JENNIFER HAYASHI DANNS was b
pool. Whilst studying for a BA (Hon
the University of Liverpool, she sp
the lap dancing industry. Jennifer worked as a Marketing
Planner for a Times 100 Best Small Company. She is
passionate about women's rights and, as a Nichiren Buddhist,
believes that every human life is precious. She lives in Rich-
mond, Surrey, with her husband Hiro.

SANDRINE LÉVÊQUE worked as Campaign Manager on
OBJECT's 'Stripping the Illusion' campaign between 2007
and 2010, which concluded successfully with the British
Government's passing of legislation that gave councils greater
control over the lap dancing industry. She now lives in France
and runs her own business, Groova, a movement, music and
well-being brand.

STRIPPED

THE BARE REALITY OF LAP DANCING

Jennifer Hayashi Danns
with Sandrine Lévêque

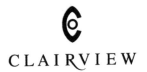

CLAIRVIEW

Clairview Books
Hillside House, The Square
Forest Row, East Sussex RH18 5ES

www.clairviewbooks.com

Published by Clairview 2011

*Apart from the named authors of this book, the names of all the contributors, as
well as the individuals they refer to, have been changed. The contributions to the
'Experiences' section have only undergone minimal editing, in order to keep the
individual voices and characters of the various pieces*

A catalogue record for this book is available from the British Library

ISBN 978 1 905570 32 4

Cover by Andrew Morgan Design
Typeset by DP Photosetting, Neath, West Glamorgan
Printed and bound by Gutenberg Press, Malta

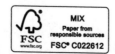

To all young women:

Love, honour and cherish yourselves. We are precious, and it is our time to shine...

'Thus I gave up myself to ruin without the least concern, and am a fair memento to all young women whose vanity prevails over their virtue: nothing was ever so stupid on both sides.'

From *Moll Flanders* by Daniel Defoe

Contents

Why I wrote this book

What is lap dancing? Whilst many people have an opinion on this subject, many are unaware of what actually happens inside the clubs themselves. The aim of this book is to give a voice to women who have direct experience of lap dancing but are often unheard, and to peel away some of the gloss surrounding this industry.

I grew up in the North West, where I attended a local comprehensive school. I did well academically but didn't really enjoy the whole experience of school. Due to my good grades I was able to attend a very good college where I completed my 'A' levels. After I finished college, I had neither the money nor the inclination to go straight to university; instead, I moved to another country to work for a season in a holiday resort. Upon returning to England I worked in several bars and clubs on minimum wages, but after a couple of years I realised that I was tired of working in poorly-paid jobs and living hand to mouth. I decided that I wanted a degree so that I could eventually start a career in business and get myself out of the minimum-wage grind.

At that time I believed that I could not afford university. I had become used to living independently. I didn't want to share a student house as I was now older than the average student, and I didn't want to do a full-time degree whilst also working a full-time job. A chance meeting introduced me to lap dancing. I met a woman who told me what she earned for two nights dancing topless in a club. It was more than I earned in a week in a regular bar. I felt frightened of doing full strip, but topless seemed less scary, and I convinced myself that this was the only way that I could go to university and achieve what I wanted in my life. Hindsight has revealed that this was not the truth; I could have taken on greater debt, or lived more humbly, but my decision was made and I began a two-year sojourn in the world of lap dancing.

I worked in one club mainly, but when the money dropped so did my personal standards. On two different occasions I went to other clubs where I performed full strip. The first time I pulled my knickers down I felt my soul fall out, but as I was convinced that money was the be-all and end-all, I worked the entire weekend. And then, months later, when money was tight again, I went and did another weekend of full strip.

My time as a lap dancer is documented in this book in greater detail; I am one of the contributors to the 'Experiences' section. Eventually the reason I stopped dancing was that I met the man who was to become my husband. Love made me realise how unhappy I was in that job, and how damaging it had become to my life. I never told anyone other than my closest friends that I was working as a lap dancer. All the people on my university course must have thought me cold, as I always refused any social invitations.

I only told my family what I was doing as one day I had a horrible thought: 'What if I was attacked one night?', or 'What if the train I took to work crashed?' – and they would have no idea where I was.

In my final year of university I had the opportunity to complete a dissertation on the subject of my choice. I was studying for a degree in business, but – with absolutely no relevance to my degree! – I based my dissertation on the lap dancing industry in the UK. Through studying for this dissertation, I found that there was little documentation of lap dancing, and that very few of the articles or pieces I found reflected my own experience and what I had seen and done. After reading my dissertation my lecturer encouraged me to explore this topic further. Although I initially received a high grade for the dissertation, when it went to the external examiners they marked it low, justifiably, as it was completely unrelated to my studies.

However, doing the dissertation gave me the confidence to believe that this industry needed to be talked about, and to an extent exposed, and that I had the ability to do it. I researched online organisations that might be interested in my dissertation, and found OBJECT. They had a campaign called 'Stripping the Illusion', which was exactly what I had been trying to achieve. I met with Sandrine Lévêque, who at that time worked for OBJECT, and so this book was born.

Nothing in life is ever all bad. Through my time as a lap dancer I made some great friends, so I was able to ask them to contribute their own experiences to this book. Sandrine, in her work with OBJECT, had also met women who either worked in or had been affected by lap dancing, and she asked them to contribute.

Working on this book has been difficult, as it has meant exposing myself as a former lap dancer. Despite my justifications to myself for being involved in this type of work, overall I have kept it a secret. In writing this, I have felt afraid of the consequences on my future career, and also the effect on my family. I am happily married, have a good relationship with my parents and family, so why not just leave all this in the past and move on with my life? This book isn't going to cure cancer, end wars, or abolish nuclear weapons, so what is the point of potentially destroying all that I have achieved so far? Who cares about lap dancers when there are so many other serious societal problems as well as atrocities taking place in the world?

The short answer is that *I* do. I know that this industry is of no value, despite all the assertions to the contrary, i.e. that it generates money for the economy, gives women confidence, allows women the opportunity to be independent and self sufficient who otherwise may be unable to work, etc. I know that I am capable of more than taking my clothes off for a living and so are all the other women in this industry. I once watched a speech given by Eve Ensler, author of *The Vagina Monologues*, in which she said that you should put into the world what you would like to have found yourself. I would like to have read this book before I began lap dancing, so I could have had some idea what I was getting myself into. I would like to give that opportunity to other young women.

All the experiences in this book are from women involved in or affected by lap dancing within the last five years. This industry is still thriving and growing. As a developed country, we must look at the causes and effects of such an industry that is entirely based on the sexual objectification of women. As I have said, there are terrible things in this world that must be addressed, and for many people lap dancing doesn't rank high on the list. But I believe that in order for change to happen in our world, people who know about things that are harming other people and causing them to suffer must stand up and share their experiences, so that we can all grow. If you know about the destruction of the environment, stand up! If you know about labour abuses, stand up! If you know about nuclear weapons, stand up! If you know about human trafficking, stand up!

Whatever you know that can help another person avoid suffering, please stand up. I know about this, so I have stood up.

In the next section of this book, women working within the industry, as well as those affected by it, are given an opportunity to express their own experience of what actually happens in lap dancing clubs, and to share the impact this thriving industry has had on their lives. Media depictions of lap dancers often fall prey to caricatured and stereotypical images of the women involved. This book aims to offer a voice to the women themselves, and thus to provide new insight and perspective into a still secretive and largely undisclosed world.

Jennifer Hayashi Danns
August 2011

Part 1
EXPERIENCES

Alicia

At just 25 years old, I have already travelled the world three times, whilst doing a degree. The first question on everyone's lips is: 'Where did you get the money to pay for it?' I do not have rich parents; no one died and left me a huge inheritance. I chose to enter the world of exotic dancing. Easy money, some might say.

My original motivations for lap dancing were not to do with money, rather to prove a point. For most of my teenage years, I had been dogged with unpopularity at school. Not feeling liked by people made me feel that I had missed out on something. I was making up for lost time in a big way, taking recreational drugs, partying, promoting club nights and podium dancing. I so strongly wanted other people my age to be envious of me. Lap dancing somehow seemed like the next logical step.

I did some research and found the number for a club, and before I knew it, I was sat face to face with the manager. He outlined the fact that working there would involve fully nude lap dancing and told me that he wanted to make sure that this was something I would be comfortable with. I replied a confident 'yes', secretly toying with my moral conscience.

I returned on a weekday, having arranged to meet with another dancer. I was shown around the club which was quite decadent, bathed in black and leopard-print with velvet dancing rooms and a looming lap dancing pole. There were bottles of Cristal and Dom Pérignon champagne in prime position behind the bar. It did not appear to be a sleazy sex establishment, but quite an upmarket venue. This provided me with some justification. I thought that only the most beautiful women would be asked to work there and felt lucky to be one of them.

As the dancer was guiding me around the workplace, she explained that a full nude dance would cost £20. I was to wear an evening dress, which specifically had to be below the knee, so as to create an air of sophistication and leave something to a man's imagination. My job would be to spend the evening persuading men to take me for a three to four minute lap dance. I would also be required to perform regular stage shows, involving the lap dancing pole.

We were expected to operate under an alias known as a stage name. I chose Alicia. The name held no significance to me. When I was working at the club, I would leave myself, the bumbling student, at the door. I was to become Alicia, the sexy, confident lap dancer. It was by this very disassociation that I would be able to cope with some of my later experiences whilst working as a lap dancer.

With my first lesson over, I hung around at the bar and ordered myself a drink, wanting to get a feel for the club and how it worked. Music began and a dancer took to the stage. She created sensual shapes and spun weightlessly around the pole. The final move consisted of an ascent to the top of the pole. There, at the precarious top, she spun upside down so that only her legs stopped her from falling. My heart flipped as she shot downwards at break-neck speed, stopping abruptly, just inches from the stage floor. The dance had been breathtaking and filled me with self doubt. I realised that I was afraid of the pole and wondered if pole dancing was an innate skill.

During the subsequent week, I would sneak downstairs, warily scouring the room to see if anyone was watching me. There, in the unnatural light, loomed the lap dancing pole: a beast that had to be tamed. I gripped it nervously with both hands and jumped up desperately trying to anchor myself with both legs, but feeling myself slowly sliding back down it, until my body slumped on the floor in a defeated heap. The dancer who had previously given me the guided tour began to show me that it did not need to be this difficult, and that the key to creating the perfect spin was where you placed your body weight. Soon, I could perform one simple spin. I had by no means mastered it and the moves that acted as fillers were awkward, but I had learnt something.

On my first night, I had borrowed a long red dress, originally worn by my house mate at her 'A' level leaving do. I wore very little make-up and compared to the other girls, plastered in make-up with dresses that screamed 'fuck me', I stuck out like an awkward sore thumb. I did not yet know how to be sexy.

I remember my first stage dance. I was thrown in at the deep end and asked to work on a night when I was supposed to be going in for another practice. Mostly, I walked around the pole and did not dare perform my new spin, just in case I fell off. Nobody commented on my less than perfect dancing, but one girl told me that I had a great pair of breasts. I don't recall the name of the man I performed my first lap dance for, nor what he looked like. I just remember feeling exposed and a tremendous sense of guilt about my boyfriend. I quickly justified it. It didn't carry the same meaning as when my boyfriend saw me naked, and it was happening to Alicia, not me. I made £40 that night.

My boyfriend had convinced himself of something along the same lines. For the most part, I felt trusted and respected. His friends thought the opposite. They would endlessly try to convince him that it was wrong to let hundreds of men see his girlfriend naked every week; they said that they wouldn't allow their girlfriends to work there. As a consequence, it became ammunition during any rows we had.

I kept my money in my bedside table drawer when I was at home. Whenever I went out, I took it all with me. This odd habit came about because I had never had this much money before, and didn't really know what to do with it. What I did know was that I didn't want to let it out of my sight for one second. Finally, when I was carrying around £100–£200 on a daily basis, my house mate convinced me to put it in the bank. Quite a risk, considering I never paid taxes.

There was a strange dynamic in the workplace at the lap dancing club. The women would get along fine in the changing rooms, like allies. Out on the floor it was a very different scenario, because we were all there to make money.

Once a dancer had initiated contact with a customer, under no circumstances could another dancer even so much as look at them, because that customer then belonged to her. If a dancer did particularly well financially, it was generally met with bitterness, rather than congratulations.

Men, male managers and male bouncers operated the club. It was blatant that they did not respect us, nor understand us on an emotional level. For the most part, the bouncers served their purpose in terms of warding off any unwanted customers, but they never stood right next to us. If a customer tried to grope us or verbally attack us during a lap dance, which they quite often did, we would have to diffuse the situation ourselves. Despite the lack of security during these situations, the manager was still happy to take expensive house fees from us and issue hefty fines for nonsensical reasons.

I always thought of the customers as vermin and, ironically, that is what they thought of me. As soon as they set foot through the door, I lost all respect for them. I would think nothing of taking advantage of the drunk ones and bleeding them dry for their money, because they deserved it. It was not a 'gentleman's' club and I failed to understand what was so gentlemanly about an intoxicated man using derogatory language towards me, pestering me for sex and getting off on my naked body. I could tolerate it because I didn't see it as a sexual act, and it was happening to Alicia, not me. Every once in a while, one of them would try to offer some understanding, asking me why I felt I had to expose my body in front of men for money, but at the end of the day, despite their show of sympathy they were still endorsing it by being in the club in the first place.

There were customers known as 'regulars'. If you had a 'regular', this meant that you had a steady flow of easy cash coming in. All a dancer would have to do was sit and endure a lonely drunk man with money, chattering away all night, and she would be presented with upwards of £500 at the end.

I worked three nights per week. I made in a week more than somebody working full-time. I had lots of free time to concentrate on studying for my degree, and did not need to go shopping at cut-price supermarkets for a single tin of beans to last me the week, like other students did. After weighing up the pros and cons, I decided that it was worth putting up with some of the negative aspects of lap dancing.

I told myself that I wasn't like the other girls. I had had a good upbringing, and was studying for a degree. I worked as a lap dancer because I wanted to and not because it was a necessity. I wasn't sexy either. I was a sexual person – I'd had boyfriends – but I was still rather naive and innocent. I realised that if I wanted to make money in this capacity, I would need to emulate the other girls. If I could get this part right, I would be quids in.

A dancer from another club brought in clothes to sell for lap dancing every now and again: rails of brightly-coloured lycra costumes and thongs. The first dress that I bought which really made me stand out was white, with latino frills. One side of it was so short it skimmed my buttocks, but the other was knee length, so this was still acceptable. I had sought the advice of another dancer, who taught me how to use eyeliner, and I began to dye my hair all the colours of the rainbow, until I finally settled on jet black. From 9 p.m. until 3 a.m. I worked solidly without a break. I steadily climbed the hierarchy, until I was the highest paid dancer there.

As the money started to roll in, my spending naturally increased. It would be fair to say that, in my youth and naivety, I was rather reckless at first. I would spend money on random items, like a pair of Chilean rats, just because I had the money to spend. I began to buy a lot of designer clothes, largely influenced by fellow lap dancers whom I looked up to. My biggest spend was in Ibiza, where I squandered £1,000 alone on a one-week stay.

My motivations for lap dancing had entirely shifted to financial gain and competition, for I had experienced the ugliness of the act itself. After I realised that my bout of reckless spending was transient and brought little meaning to why I was lap dancing, I began to channel my wages into more positive things, like a plane ticket for my boyfriend to go and visit his parents in Spain, and a trip to Brazil, so that I could teach English for two months.

There was a significant shift at the club with the arrival of a group of new girls. They had a clear leader, a blonde girl, whose name I cannot remember. She stood in the centre of the changing rooms with a group of girls with whom she had not previously met, and unashamedly proclaimed that she had an amazing pussy, inviting everyone to see for themselves. She spoke of her boyfriend's imprisonment, like it was something to be proud of. She instantly shot to popularity, partly because of her unreservedness, but mainly because other dancers were intimidated by her.

Before this time, lap dancers adhered to strict rules. You had to remain three feet away from the customer, and under no circumstances could you spread your legs after you had taken off your thong. Ignoring these rules was seen as 'dirty dancing', and a 'dirty lap dancer' would be dogged by rumours of prostitution. The new group of girls did not adhere to these rules. They would slide down customers and place their nipples in the customer's mouths, engage in sexual contact with other lap dancers, and graphically spread their legs. Strangely they were not met with the same icy reception as other lap dancers who sunk to this level would usually have received. It was inevitable that the wrong people would eventually find out about the illegal activity, but both the staff and the other lap dancers allowed it to go on.

The rules shifted. If dancers wanted to stay on top of their game, they would have to adhere to these new rules. It was simple. The customers were visiting the club for a sexual release. If some lap dancers were offering more, they were the lap dancers they would go for. The customers grew more disrespectful, asking us why we were not offering the same services as the other girls. I admit that for a while I would spread my legs. Although my moral compass drew the line at physical contact, which would blur the lines with prostitution, I still look back upon this time with deep regret. I felt I had to do it.

I stayed on top, partly because I was smart and would use my powers of persuasion, and partly because the men could see literally everything. This didn't go unnoticed by the new group of girls, and they began to spread malicious rumours. They had to get rid of the competition.

One night the new girl approached me outside of work, in a nightclub, whilst I was out with my friends. She confessed that she was a heroin addict and that she had heard I was too. I recoiled in horror. Is that what people thought of me? I was not the same as her, or was I, in some way? I had to convince myself again that Alicia was a character I was playing, not really me, and that it was worth people viewing me this way for the money I was making.

Back at work, the new group of girls gradually started to turn other lap dancers against me, and they would give the bouncers, the very people that were meant to protect me, money to lie about my lap dances to the managers. I was branded a 'dirty dancer' and a drug addict, so it was no surprise to me that when undercover police found out about the illegal practice of the dirty dancing, the club insisted that 'it must have been Alicia'.

On the back of the police investigation, I was one of the first to lose my job. It had been two years. It hit me all at once, and I felt a powerful hurt and humiliation. Around this time, I also split up with my boyfriend. His friends nagged away at him, because they thought he deserved better. During my subsequent years as a lap dancer I had only one night stands, just as meaningless as the lap dances I performed. The truth was, no man wanted a girl whom everyone else could share intimately. Where would be the exclusivity in that?

I went on to a short-lived job at another lap dancing club. It was in the middle of an industrial estate and was a somewhat shabby establishment. In a way, I admired the honesty of that. It wasn't pretending to be something that it wasn't. I was relieved that there were rules there, and that I did not have to lower myself to earn my place. Three feet away, no floor work at all, and definitely no spreading of legs when the thong was removed.

This would all have been fine if it wasn't for the other lap dancers. They were convinced that, again, I was a 'dirty dancer', and questioned my earnings; so much so that they had me watched by the bouncers. They found nothing untoward. Yet, still, I experienced violent threats. They wanted me out. One evening, I found the inside of my bag had been splattered with wine. I ignored it and made to leave, but one of the dancers tripped me up. Another blocked the door. 'Where do you think you're going?' I mustered up all my energy and screamed: 'Move out of my fucking way!' They had never experienced such aggression from me, neither had I. Something clicked. I would have to toughen up if I was going to make it in this world. She moved out of my way without hesitation. I walked out of that club, and never returned.

The next club in which I worked was different. This period

marked a substantial turning point. Instead of territorial gangs, the dancers were normal women who were very much together as a group, in that they supported each other, and any disagreements were sorted out amicably. I was immediately embraced within their community. I was not earning the same money as I was at the first club, but it was still enough to live comfortably and to save for my second trip to America. I worked hard and was on top of my game, but the fundamental difference was that this time I was actually getting praise for it. I received compliments from the other dancers, instead of jealousy and hatred. I became affectionately known by the owner and manageress as the 'little star' and a 'grafter'. They would grab my hand, lead me over to customers and proudly explain: 'This is the best girl here'.

I am certain that none of the girls were prostitutes and drugs were never an issue at this club. This would not be tolerated. Any dancers that came to work for the club with a bad attitude were ignored, and they swiftly left. The idea of an atmosphere other than harmony was never entertained. Another positive effect of this was you knew the other dancers would not hear a bad word said against you. One of the bitches that had got me sacked from the other club came to work there and attempted to resurface the old rumours. The other dancers told her straight that her behaviour was unacceptable, and she soon left.

For the first time, I could actually say that I had allies, even friends, within the workplace. However, our relationship was still a bit odd. I would go out with them socially on numerous occasions. At times, the nights out would turn rough; they would get into physical fights. I could do nothing but stand back. I knew that if it was me fighting, the other dancers would defend me, but I had never been in a fight in my life, and I was too afraid to jump in.

I worked there quite happily for two years. Towards the end of these two years there was a dramatic downfall, but this was in no way the fault of the club. It wasn't even a gradual decline. One day, men just stopped visiting the club and it was dead. Earnings dried up, no matter how much promotional work we did around the city centre. Before, we had lived comfortably. Now it was touch and go as to whether we would make enough money to pay the rent.

Looking back, I am repulsed with how I dealt with this decline. The bottom line was simply this: the large amounts of money we were getting paid were the only justification for sharing my body with the men that walked through the doors of the club each night. If the money was taken away, then so too was a great deal of my self-worth. I began to drink heavily on work nights, which is something I had never done before. When I was drunk, I would complain loudly that I should have been getting paid. There was general unrest amongst the dancers, but I was one of the few who took it hard.

The bouncers, afraid for their jobs as the club faded, all resigned *en masse*. New security was hired. We quickly discovered that they were more concerned with play fighting amongst themselves and nipping outside for extended cigarette breaks, than with providing safety for the dancers.

As a consequence we would have to diffuse any sexual or verbal confrontation ourselves. With the lack of money and the lack of security, I could feel an anger burning inside of me.

On one occasion a customer took it a step too far. I was accustomed to verbal abuse and constant propositions – that, I had learned to handle. Usually, I could see a man's hands rising up to grip my waist from a mile off. I was dancing as normal, when the customer pushed his hand between my legs. I darted quickly away from him, feeling violated and physically sick. I looked around me and there were no bouncers present to intercept and help me. I decided I would have to take care of the matter myself, so I slapped him hard across the face.

Despite having notified the bouncers of the incident, I still saw the customer drinking with his friends at the club. I could see him laughing at me, probably discussing the act that he had gotten away with to his friends, like I was nothing but an object. I marched up to him and demanded that he leave the club. When he laughed I came out with the most insulting thing I could muster. I told him to fuck off back to Pakistan. I am mortified that I said this, as I'm not racist. I just wanted him to feel as awful as he had just made me feel. My anger and frustration had totally warped my personality.

I could feel everyone's eyes upon me, shocked at what had come out of my mouth. The manageress told me she wanted me to leave the club straight away. I probably could have grovelled and got my job back, as I knew I had enough of a presence there, but it wasn't worth it. It was no longer a safe place to work, and there were no longer any financial rewards.

By this time, I was saving up for a six-month round-the-world trip. I began to work in Blackpool, in a weird little place that was an absolute gold mine for lap dancers for one reason only. It was the capital of stag dos. That meant new men would be visiting the club every week who had never previously laid eyes on you. 'Regulars', who had seen it all before and were too bored to pay anymore, were now a thing of the past.

I was no stranger to late night shifts, but my new hours were ridiculous. I would work 14-hour shifts in six inch stilettos, often without a break. I could not sleep at night because of the agonising pain in my feet, but the money made it worth it.

The club was very light-hearted in its approach to the stags. The men would enter the club wearing some sort of lavish, ridiculous costume. I did not like the stage shows. These were aimed to surprise the stag into an act of humiliation on the main stage. The stag would be tied up, whipped, led around the stage and made to bark like a dog, and would finally have the names of two dancers emblazoned across his chest in permanent marker. I actually regarded the act as more humiliating for the dancers, and saw it as a way for the men to see the breasts of the dancers for free, which defeated the object of individual, paid-for, lap dances. For these reasons, I refused to do stage shows.

I finished my degree and, when I set off on my six-month trip, I met my fiancé. This seemed like a natural time to end my stint in the world of exotic dancing. I wanted to begin my career, and I loved a man so much that I wanted to be his and his alone. I don't know if I ever will reach a decision on what to make of my experiences as a lap dancer. On the one hand, I think I did lose my innocence. I chose to put myself in a world in which I have questioned my personal morals. Sometimes, it makes me feel ashamed, and I feel that my fiancé deserves someone who hasn't been tainted so much. On the other hand, my eyes are open, I feel stronger, and the financial gain has presented me with opportunities beyond my wildest dreams. One thing is crystal clear: that lap dancing has had a deep effect on my life.

Topaz

I began lap dancing in a club in Blackpool. The motivation to begin dancing is now somewhat of a cliché: I wanted to go to university and I could not afford to, although with hindsight — that wonderful phenomenon — I now question if this was true. I could have worked full time in a low-paid job or lived at home with my parents, but I didn't want to. I wanted what I perceived others to have: an independent home and disposable income. I fell hook, line and sinker for the hard-sell of consumerism. I had chosen my path.

In a hairdresser's I met a young woman who disclosed that she was a lap dancer. My impression of lap dancers up to that point was that they were all slags who loved showing their bodies to men and got off on it, and also that they only did it because they were too stupid to do anything else. This girl, however, was a mother: very beautiful, with brown hair, tall and looked like a model; not bleach blond with massive fake tits. She encouraged me to try it for one night and if I did not like it I could just leave.

At that time I was not particularly over-confident or, the other extreme, very shy. I liked my body the same way other girls do; sometimes I felt fat, other times I felt great. The club in Blackpool was just a topless club, so when you danced you stripped to your knickers. I rationalised that I go topless on a beach so what is the difference? At least I would be getting paid for men ogling at me this way. I had previously worked in ordinary bars, and the higher I hoisted my bust in a low cut top, the more tips I would earn, so I thought, fuck it! — may as well just get over any morals I have. I had been a form of stripper for years in ordinary bars, using my body to my advantage to get tips from male customers.

The first time I walked into the club my impression was that it was 'classy'. An older blonde woman, who looked like a madam from a saloon in old Western films, ran the club. New dancers are supposed to audition, which involves performing a pole dance in the centre of the club in front of the manager (the blonde madam!) and also all the other dancers who work there. I was shitting myself because I had never ever swung round a pole in my life. When the manager saw me she said that I could start to work straight away and did not need to audition, as I was pretty and looked good and she was certain I would be great for the club. She asked me what my stage name was, and I just looked at her blankly. 'Every girl has a glamorous name.' 'Like what?', I asked. 'Like Crystal, or Sapphire.' So I, in a brain fart that I would live to regret, said: 'Well my birth stone is Topaz.' 'Topaz!', she screeched back at me. 'That's perfect, fabulous. Topaz go and get ready.'

From then I was no more, Topaz was born.

The new name thing is weird and far from glamorous. From then on I would introduce myself as Topaz to the customers, and one of two things always happened:

Number 1/ the nice ones, or the ones who get bang into the whole lap dancing role play thing, would say something on the lines of: 'That's a beautiful name ... very exotic ... is that a name from your country?' Now I can just about forgive that. I am British, but I am mixed race, so I guess they could delude themselves into believing that they were getting a dance from a foreign girl, except for the fact that I had a 24-year-old strong Liverpudlian accent that I made no attempt to hide. So, why the fuck they believed I was Topaz from a far-away exotic land with a voice like Steven Gerrard, I don't know.

Number 2/ the weird ones, or the ones who are paranoid, would say: 'There is no fucking way that is your name ... tell me your real name ... I am not going to stalk you or anything', which had the immediate effect of making me think they would stalk me and possibly chop me up and put my head in the freezer. So then I would say: 'OK, my real name is Natalie' (my real name is not Natalie!), and they would then think they were my best mate for life, and that I had just disclosed my deepest darkest secret to them.

Anyway, I hit the floor the first night as Topaz. The girl I had met in the hairdresser's took me under her wing and led me to the private room where she gave me a lap dance to show me what I needed to do. Then she asked me to give her a lap dance, throughout which she gave a running commentary of what was right and wrong, and more so what was sexy and what was just plain scary.

It is odd to dance for a girl. Later on in my foray into lap dancing, I danced for a lot of female customers who often came in with their partners, and it was always a disconcerting experience, no matter how many times I did it. Women really,

really look at your body, and the dance you do for a man feels so stupid when you perform it for a woman. Squeezing my boobs in some woman's face is one of the times I was grateful for the stupid name, so I could pretend to be someone else for the three minutes and I had to just convince myself in my head that I was not doing this for a tenner.

It's worse dancing for a couple in a private room. It is just wrong and feels so intimate and intense. You know that they are there to 'spice up' their relationship, and you are some kind of tool for them to achieve that. I really had to mentally switch off, and at times it was so intense I would feel physically sick. Dances such as those were when I would feel a bit like a sex worker rather than an 'entertainer'.

Back to the first night: my first dance was for an unattractive, overweight middle-aged man who was apparently a regular in the club. I forgot to take my dress off and had to dance for him again. After the dance, in which I stripped to my knickers, I asked him what he thought, and he said I was shit. I apologised and told him that he was my first ever dance. He looked mortified, said sorry to me, gave me an extra £20 and bought me a drink, then gave me guidance on how to dance better. All the way through his pep talk I thought, What a prick!

After this I got progressively better. At that time I did not realise that lap dancing had hit an earning peak and had begun to decline. On average, in the beginning I would earn about £250 to £400 a night after paying my house fee of £60 to £80. This to me was great, and more than I would earn working all week in a normal bar. The other girls, after an initial spell of mistrust, defensiveness and bitchiness, began to accept me, and for a time lap dancing was great, and a job that I thought I enjoyed. I felt sexy and confident in work, and felt part of a team with the other girls. The manager really liked me and was always complementary to me and fair. The customers were a mixed bag, but in the majority they were nice and generous with buying drinks and tipping, after having already paid £10 for a private dance.

As in any job there were good nights and bad, but overall the first six months to a year were good, and I had earned enough money to confidently start university, and could afford to live in my own apartment and not go into halls of residence. However, nothing lasts forever, and after a while the decline in lap dancing, and the change in the outside world, began to show.

In Blackpool lots of other rival clubs began to open, and another major shift was that the female owner and manager left and was replaced by a man. A woman understands the nature of lap dancing from a female perspective, whereas a man often perceives the dancers very differently, usually from the wider society perspective that we are all glorified sluts. The club rapidly transformed from the classy, sexy, relaxed lap dancing club to a stripping club, where it seemed almost anything went.

The original manager would only allow a specific number of girls per night to meet demand, so that we would all have a fair chance at earning money. Also, she intentionally chose the girls working to ensure a range of choice for the men, so there were blondes, brunettes, older girls, younger girls, slim girls, bigger girls, etc. My place was assured as I was one of the few black girls, and at one time the only black girl. At the time this process seemed normal but with hindsight it is dehumanising and basically a kind of cattle market. Men would come in and ask the manager if she had any black girls, and I would be wheeled over like a prize cow.

The strange thing about lap dancing is how things that would be unacceptable in real life become normal in the club. Even before the shift from good place to work to awful, the things happening during the 'good' period are strange to think about now.

During the good times, the range of dances on offer was:

A dance in the open club at the customer's seat (where everyone else in the club can see you dancing topless): £5.

A private one-to-one dance (in a private room away from the club floor, but with other dancers in the same room): £10.

A girl-on-girl dance (two girls dancing for one customer in the private room): £20 (£10 per girl).

A lesbian show (either in the private room or on the main stage in the club): £40 (£20 per girl).

The £5 dance was avoided wherever possible, as you could not move properly. All the other customers watching could see you dancing badly, and also could see you topless without actually paying anything; so in terms of PR it was a bad move, and every girl avoided this like the plague. But there was always one, usually a new girl that no one had explained it to, who would do a £5 dance, then all the fuckers would want one.

The private one-on-one dance was everyone's bread and butter, and the trick was to try and get them to stay in there as long as possible and have multiple dances at £10 each. The manipulative trick to this was to remain topless, lean over and whisper in their ear: 'Would you like me to carry on?', to which any red-blooded man would pant, 'Yes!', whether they could afford it or not. This is one of the things that I would never have dreamed I would do, but I did because it is so normal in lap dancing.

The girl-on-girl dance was risky as you could potentially make more money dancing on your own, and if the girl was a bitch she could, and would, steal your customer. Again, despite my assertions of being part of a team, it was still normal to stab each other in the back for a dance, and ultimately for a tenner.

The lesbian shows are possibly the worst part of the whole dancing experience, and to me the greatest justification that lap dancing is part of the sex industry. Again, still considering the 'good' times of my experience dancing, the lesbian show could be, and usually was, awful. The lesbian show in the private room involved me and probably someone I would call a friend fondling each other and pretending to be lesbians in front of a fully-clothed man. As sick as it was to do this, with a friend it was far safer than dancing with another girl.

I would do lesbian dances when the amount I had earned was not enough, or on a slow night, even though I hated them. The lesbian show was for me a major indicator of how my personal morals were beginning to slip significantly. The reason it was safer to perform such a dance with a friend was that you would know each other's limits. To me, it was £20; £20 does not condone a full-on soft porn show, which was the level other girls took it to. In one instance I danced with another girl, and she grabbed my boobs, put my nipples in her mouth, and kissed me full on the mouth. She then tried to lick my vagina through my knickers. The whole experience made me feel sick and dirty, and I really wanted to hit her for what she had done. After this I would choose the girls carefully to dance with, and whenever possible refused to do a lesbian show.

Another bizarre phenomenon, during what I am increasingly realising may *not* have been such a good time, was girls selling their knickers to customers. Men would often ask me if they could buy my knickers, to which my answer was always no. However, I know other girls actually brought in spare pairs of knickers to sell to customers. One girl I saw 'soiled' the knickers with baby lotion to look like she had worn them, and sold them to a customer for £20. As shocking as some of this may sound, this was normal in 'classy' lap dancing, and a part of the job that over time you just learned to accept. In comparison to the events that occurred under the new manager, these events are relatively tame.

Under the new manager the club turned into a horrible, sleazy, vile place to work. The first major change was new girls. These girls would grind on customers' laps, which serves the purpose of masturbating a customer with their arse. They would pull their knickers to the side and flash their vagina to the customer. They would simulate and in some cases actually masturbate themselves in front of the customer. There were a lot of rumours that they were having sex and performing sex acts on the manager and the new male owner. They would accept dances for drugs, such as cocaine, instead of money. They would make arrangements to meet customers after work. In the lesbian shows they would masturbate each other, allow customers to touch them, kiss each other and customers. All for the same price as I was charging for a no-contact, topless, £10 lap dance.

There was no way to compete with this, so I got increasingly drunk. All the way through dancing I had used alcohol, to the point that I could not work without a drink. At this point I began to abuse alcohol as I was so upset with how the club had become. I would not engage in any of that sexual activity for a dance, so — as in the beginning of my dancing career — I was told by customers that my dance was shit because I was not touching myself or them. It was unbearable, and mentally difficult to deal with.

Other girls, who started out as good girls, would quickly descend to the level of animals and compete with other girls by out-filthing each other. The customers began to turn and would say awful, awful things to the girls. One example of this was a man who said to me: 'You best make this dance worth my while.' I asked him what he meant and he said: 'You best be the dirtiest one in here.' I told him I wasn't, and he said: 'Well, if you are not going to finger yourself I am not giving you a tenner.' To which I told him to fuck off and die. He just walked off and found a girl who would do that.

I began to frequently have such arguments with the customers. They would touch me and grab me, and one even bit me during a dance. I did not feel safe. I also felt ashamed to be working in the club and thought to myself that if someone attacked me in here, or when I walked home, no court would prosecute the attacker. People would say that I deserved it. I hated myself and everyone else in there, but felt trapped as, by this point, I was hardly making any money as I would not dance the way the dirty girls were. I frequently was only making enough to cover the house fee, train ticket and bed-and-breakfast, with no extra profit for myself.

Increasingly, rather than getting dances, I was making customers buy me a drink instead, and I am ashamed to admit that often I would be so drunk that I would lose my dancing money, fight with other girls and customers, and not remember getting back home. It was hell — a hell that I had chosen to place myself in. One night I had a drunken fight with the disgusting new manager, and he sacked me for calling him a twat. Even after this I went back, and I cannot honestly say why. Maybe one night in a month I would make some money, and I convinced myself that it would get better but it never did.

Finally, I left after two years and, because of the way lap dancing clubs are now, would never ever go back. At the end it was dehumanising, soul destroying, and filled with desperation. Desperate girls trying to make £100 a night however they could, and thinking that was good money. Desperate girls selling their souls for a part in this 'glamorous' industry. Desperate girls thinking that lap dancing is about flashing their vagina and explicitly simulating sex. All that was ever fun and could have been called harmless had gone. There is no talent involved in lap dancing any more, and the willingness for sexual degradation needed to compete in this industry now is truly frightening.

It is strange to talk about all of this since I have finished dancing and moved on with my life. Many parts of my time in dancing are difficult to talk about. Often if someone asked about my experience as a dancer I have responded with a socially acceptable answer, and simply asserted that I enjoyed dancing, that I made a lot of money, but in the end dancing was not for me. This explanation in no way conveyed the extremity of emotion and mental distress I experienced as a dancer, and in no way conveys the sexual degradation and humiliation I experienced and observed during my short dancing career. I am also able to acknowledge the naivety out of which I began dancing, as initially I did not associate myself or my actions with the sex industry. Now I would accept that I was part of the sex industry, especially towards the latter stages of my experience, and although I did not personally engage in any sexual activities within the club, by association with the other dancers who were displaying explicit sexual behaviour, and my acceptance of employment in the same club, I could be labelled as a sex worker, which I find very upsetting. I believe that my experience is reflective of young women now, who begin lap dancing perceiving it to be glamorous, and with the expectation of earning vast amounts of money, but who will receive a shock and have to face the decision as to whether this is the industry they truly want to be involved in.

Journalist

Ask any journalist and they will tell you that it's impossible to close your notebook at night and forget about the story you're working on. It's also impossible to finish a story and hold the same opinion on it as you did when you started. If your opinion hasn't changed, then either it wasn't a story in the first place, or you haven't been talking to the right people. And most journalists will readily admit that in the time they're researching a story, they become neurotically obsessed by it. It becomes a compulsion to tell anyone who'll listen every new detail you've uncovered, and to explain how it has confounded your expectations. That's how you spot a good story – it's one you have to tell.

But some stories keep on bothering you long after they rightfully should, because you feel that you haven't put your point across well enough, or it hasn't been properly understood. And that, for a journalist, is the worst feeling you can get – that somehow, you haven't told the truth.

This, for me, is that story.

In early 2008 I was asked to look into lap dancing for a current affairs television show. At that time it was rapidly becoming a big deal. In just over three years, the number of lap dancing clubs in the UK had doubled from 150 to over 300, spreading out from the murkier parts of city centres to unremarkable small towns in the provinces – and that hadn't gone unnoticed. Around the UK, local residents' groups were coming together to decry the fact that behind closed doors on their High Streets, women in various states of undress were writhing around in front of fully clothed men.

At that point I was the classic liberal in the lap dancing debate. The office I worked in was located on the backstreets of central Manchester, close to a strip club that had a near legendary reputation amongst Mancunian men, and seemed to be open 24 hours a day. Post smoking-ban, the dancers would stand outside the entrance at nine in the morning, swathed in dressing gowns and toking deeply on their cigarettes. They didn't look glamorous, or sleazy, or oppressed. If anything, they looked cold – but at least they were always laughing, which is more than you can say about the average till-girl in a supermarket. I talked with a male friend who occasionally went to the club; not to buy a lap dance, apparently, but just to have a drink and a chat with the girls. 'I just walk in and start a conversation with them and they love it', he told me. 'It's not all about sex.'

I was also reading stories, surfacing periodically in the weekend tabloid supplements, about the students making a mint working part-time as lap dancers. They described it as though it were the epitome of empowerment – working a couple of nights a week, getting paid more than some women do in a full-time job, and leaving university without debt. If lap dancing was working out for these women, then why should it be an issue that bothered me?

The first thing I did was to get on the phone to OBJECT, a

feminist pressure group who reckoned they had got to the bottom of why the clubs had suddenly multiplied. Their research revealed that a deeply buried clause in the Licensing Act — that notorious piece of New Labour legislation which brought in 24-hour drinking — had grouped lap dancing clubs together with other entertainment venues into a 'one size fits all' licensing category. That meant that suddenly, in the eyes of the law, lap dancing clubs were no different to karaoke bars, kebab houses or roller discos. And that in turn meant that it was a lot easier — and a lot cheaper — for the clubs to get licenses.

OBJECT's research was watertight and it was a good story. But they were campaigning against the clubs on the grounds that their spread was symptomatic of society's increasing objectification of women. But that didn't gel with what I had read about the dancers who paid for their degrees by working in the clubs. Let's face it, they had left university owing nothing whilst I was saddled with thousands of pounds worth of debt — so who was more oppressed? In short, OBJECT seemed to be letting their values get in the way of reasoned argument. This was a licensing issue, but I could see no reason why it should be a feminist one.

I started trying to talk to the dancers outside the club on my way to work. They were friendly enough, but none of them were about to divulge any intimate details of their profession. 'How do I know you're not going to put this on telly?' asked one.

Meanwhile, the commissioners had been considering the

story. As well as critiquing the Licensing Act, they also wanted us to employ that old staple of current affairs TV – the undercover camera. They wanted to show that despite being licensed as entertainment venues, some of the clubs were offering anything but your average night out; essentially they wanted to find out if there was sex for sale. But in order to film secretly inside the clubs, we first had to find evidence that there was something to film. The dancers I had spoken to certainly weren't going to tell me anything, so I began exploring other sources. I scoured internet forums and chat rooms for any snippets of evidence about what was going on in the clubs. And I set about meeting as many dancers as I could.

Sarah was the first. She had posted a spirited response to an online article about the Fawcett Society's condemnation of the growing corporate culture of lap dancing – top end firms taking their clients to strip clubs to secure business deals. What was interesting was that she argued that the licensing of lap dancing clubs should be more restrictive; that if fewer clubs were able to open then the industry might be forced to smarten up its image. She also claimed that most of the dancers loved their work, and were not forced into it through financial circumstances. What Sarah was saying reconfirmed everything I'd originally thought about OBJECT – that they were putting words into the mouths of women who could speak very well for themselves, and who certainly didn't need anyone campaigning on their behalf. I wanted to meet Sarah myself and find out more about her world, so I tracked her down through Facebook and sent her a message explaining what I was doing. A couple of days later I received a reply – she would be happy to meet up for a chat.

We met in a pub in a greying Northern town on a Tuesday lunchtime. She was petite, dark haired, strikingly pretty and dressed like a modern celebrity in a floral dress and knee high boots. I had imagined her to be perma-tanned and enhanced, but she looked nothing like the pneumatic Amazonian lap dancers you see in music videos. She was also supremely self possessed. As we walked around the corner to another pub that she suggested would be quieter and easier to talk in, I felt slightly ashamed of my preconceptions and positively scruffy in her company. I wondered whether it was her lap dancing night job that had given her such poise.

Sarah had begun working as a lap dancer in her home town, down south. She wanted to be a graphic designer and was planning to start a university course in the autumn. The lap dancing was a way of making money in the meantime. She described how a friend who worked as a dancer had suggested that she give it a go. 'I've never been shy or ashamed of my body so I thought, why not? It's a good way of making money. Everyone there knows it's just a bit of fun. It's a performance. It's also really good exercise.'

Sarah certainly didn't seem subjugated; but as we continued talking, I began to pick up cracks in her argument. If the job was so good, then why did the clubs need tighter regulation?

'At the moment, any Tom, Dick or Harry can set up a lap

dancing club. All the ones I've worked in have been fine, but some of them are run by real gangsters. People who don't give a shit about the women working for them.'

'In what way?'

'Well in every club the dancers are self-employed. You pay for your spot on the floor and then you earn back the money by doing dances. The more dances you do, the more money you make. Now in some clubs they'll take a percentage of your earnings, sometimes as much as 50 per cent. So however hard you work, you're always making money for the club. I'll only work in the ones where they take a set amount from you for each shift.'

'And how much is that?'

'It varies ... but anything up to £80.'

I thought about that for a moment. That meant that a dancer would be £80 down before she'd begun her shift – a lot of money if you're not going to see it again. £80 was certainly more than I was making in a day. I asked Sarah whether any of the dancers ever failed to make their money back.

'Well I never have,' she replied, 'but I suppose some do. You've just got to make sure that the men want dances from you. It's a marketplace.'

'In that case, do any of the dancers offer more than just lap dances?'

Sarah shook her head violently. 'No. Definitely not. At least not in any of the clubs I've worked in.'

Meeting Sarah left me slightly uneasy. On the surface she

was the poster girl for the empowered lap dancer; making good money, having fun. But what she had told me about the way the clubs employed their dancers suggested that there were others out there who did not have it quite so good. As we said our goodbyes I asked her why she'd moved up north. 'I came up here with my boyfriend', she said. 'We met down south but he's a Northerner and he wanted to come back home.'

'Doesn't he mind that you strip for other men?'

'Oh no!' she said breezily. 'He likes it. He brings his mates into the club to show me off.'

As she left to relax before her shift, I wondered just how much money she could really be making — and how much fun she was really having — in a depressed industrial town that had never really recovered from the last recession before being plunged into this one.

Back in the office I had found a website carrying reviews for the club around the corner. The consensus seemed to be that the club was a good one: the girls were 'stunning', the dances were cheap, and the atmosphere was laid back. But some reviewers weren't so generous. One customer said that the girl who gave him a dance needed to 'drink more water and get to the gym'. Another intoned that the club was only good if you were into cellulite. Internally I seethed at the baseness of it and wondered just how fit and toned those punters were themselves. But thinking about it more, I reasoned that these women's bodies were commodities like anything else. The men were paying for them, and they were entitled to rate them as anything else they'd spent their hard-earned cash on. As Sarah had explained, it was a marketplace. Still, I couldn't shake the feeling that there was something wrong with a man sizing up a woman in such a literal way. If someone had written that about me on the internet, I'd be livid.

For the purposes of our undercover filming the web was turning out to be little help. There is an online community for almost everyone, from prostitutes to airline pilots, but there seemed to be none for lap dancers. It was odd – this was a growing and increasingly acceptable industry after all. Everyone did it, didn't they? Major lap dancing clubs had welcomed celebrities, and even royalty had been rumoured to enjoy the company of a lap dancer or two. So why weren't people talking about it online? The few bits of testimony I did find were from scattered sources like student forums and private blogs. But there were few suggestions that you could buy anything more than a dance in any of the clubs, so we hired a male journalist to go in and see for himself. As he embarked on a grand lap dancing tour of the UK, I turned my attention back to the dancers. I was told to find one who would talk on screen about the nature of the job and what went on inside the clubs. Sarah, for all her eulogising, was not prepared to do that.

Without the aid of the internet I tried other methods to find my dancers. I placed an advert in the back of *The Stage*, the industry magazine for actors and performers, asking for current and former dancers who would be willing to contribute to a documentary about the rise of lap dancing. I put the same ad in *The Metro*, expecting to hear from countless more women like Sarah; but I heard nothing. I rang around the editors of student newspapers, many of whom had run stories about the women who were paying their way through university by lap dancing, but none of them could put me in touch with anyone. In desperation I went back to the forums and chat rooms to see if there was anyone I had overlooked in my original research. I got a couple of initial responses, but never got near anyone who was willing to take part in the programme.

So I did the last thing I wanted to do – I went back to OBJECT and asked if they were in contact with any lap dancers who might be willing to speak to me. I felt I was carrying out flawed research; OBJECT clearly had an agenda to push, and that would be reflected in the women they'd put me in touch with. But at that stage I had been left with few options, so I took a train down to London to meet Karen, a former lap dancer who was working with OBJECT on their campaign.

The Shoreditch bar where we arranged to meet was far removed from the chain pub where I'd met Sarah – and Karen herself was completely different too. Whereas Sarah oozed confidence, Karen withered into herself as we talked. Like Sarah she was petite and pretty, but I just couldn't imagine this woman taking her clothes off for money. She seemed so fragile and birdlike that I couldn't even imagine her working as a barmaid let alone taking on critical punters like the ones I'd encountered on the internet. On top of that she was obviously an intellectual – not just bright like Sarah – but truly deep thinking. She told me she was writing a play.

'It took me a long time to recover from my experiences as a lap dancer', Karen said. 'It took a long time before I could look at men as anything other than punters. Working in that industry distorts your perception of normal relationships.'

Karen had worked for a well-known lap dancing chain that operated clubs around London, and she had started because she needed the money. 'I was unemployed and I had rent and bills to pay, and it seemed like an easy way to get myself out of a mess.'

The company she'd worked for was meant to be one of the reputable ones, well run, above board, a respectable night out, a good place to work. But the picture Karen painted was very different.

'If the managers liked you then you'd be put in one of the central clubs, where all the lawyers and businessmen and city boys go. That's where you can make real money. But it's also where you find more than just lap dancing, if you know what I mean. It's a competitive environment, not a very nice environment. They always have more girls working than they actually need. So loads of the dancers get pissed or wasted on coke before their shift so that they lower their inhibitions and perform better.'

This sounded so different to the light-hearted theatrical environment that Sarah had described, but I had little doubt that Karen was telling the truth. She seemed to have been both physically and mentally affected by her time as a lap dancer. I asked why she hadn't raised her concerns with the managers.

'The people who run these clubs, they're not nice people. They're scary. From time to time these shadowy figures would come in, and you just knew that they were the people in charge of it all. I never wanted to rock the boat.'

Meeting Karen jolted my thought processes, and I began to question my *laissez-faire* attitude to lap dancing. This wasn't just about a women's right to use her body to make money, it was also about working conditions and employment issues. If what Karen was saying was right, then dancers were working in environments which encouraged them to compete in how far they'd go in their dances, and added an edge of desperation by ensuring that they started every shift owing money to the club. 'What girls going into the industry don't realise is that it's actually far from easy', she told me.

Suddenly, all my other efforts to track down dancers began to yield results. Within a week I received two phone calls from former dancers who had seen my ad in *The Stage* – and what they had to say confirmed the story Karen had told. These were women who had gone into dancing young, in their late teens and early twenties, lured by the promise of serious cash and the whiff of glamour. One had bought a house off the back of the money she'd made as a dancer back in the 1990s.

'That was when lap dancing clubs were rare and exclusive', she said. 'All of the customers were businessmen and they all spent a lot of money.'

I asked if it was still possible to earn that kind of cash and she laughed derisively. 'Anyone can be a lap dancer now', she snorted down the phone. 'When I started, you had to have the body, the personality and the wit to do it. The men I used to dance for weren't stupid, and they didn't want to spend the evening with a woman who was stupid either. They wanted a woman who looked good and who was clever enough to stroke their ego. They paid good money to get the best.'

Our undercover reporter was coming back with stories of clubs where a lap dance could be bought for £5. I asked her what the going rate was for a lap dance in London in the '90s. 'Put it this way', she told me, 'there was one night when I walked out of that club with over £2000 in my pocket. At £5 a time, that would have been a lot of lap dances. Girls now might go into lap dancing thinking they're going to make the kind of money I used to make, but in reality they're often lucky if they end up on the minimum wage.'

Another woman had given up working in the clubs to become a pole dancing teacher. Like Karen she had little that was positive to say about her time as a dancer. 'It's screwed up my view of men', she told me. 'Every time I see a man now, I just see him as a punter. There's only so many bad experiences you can have before you start hating them all.'

I asked her what she meant by 'bad experiences'. 'You know … men grabbing you or insulting you, or just being scary. Every time I left the club after a shift I wondered if one of them was going to attack me as I walked to my car. The bouncers are meant to look after you but they can't watch everyone all the time.'

So why was she now working as a pole dancing teacher, if her experiences had been so bad?

'I can't do anything else', she sighed. 'I started in that job when I was 19, and for a few years the going was good. I was earning a decent living, way better than anything I could earn working in a shop or a bar. But by the time I realised how much it was fucking me up, it was too late. I was in my late 20s, trained for nothing, and with no other work experience behind me. I've applied for different jobs but I always get the same response. They want to know what I've been doing with myself for the past decade. I'm certainly not going to tell them I've been taking my clothes off for money.'

The programme's transmission date was pulling closer, and I still hadn't found any dancers who would tell the camera what they had told me in private. But our undercover filming was bringing results. At clubs around the country dancers were making it clear to our reporter that if he had the money, then sex was on offer. At one London club there even appeared to be a back room which the dancers specifically used as a brothel. In other clubs, dancers told him they could come back to his hotel room, or get a 'dirtier dance'. Our footage demolished the lie that lap dancing was a leisure pursuit like any other.

By the time I met Jackie, a former dancer who was helping OBJECT with their campaign, I was desperate to make some sort of sense of it all. I was grappling with so many different stories, all of them told so sincerely, that I was finding it difficult to reconcile them. How could Sarah and Karen think so differently? I couldn't accept that it was just because they were so different as people; they were both intelligent women who could surely go beyond their own experiences to look at the wider picture of lap dancing. Why was it apparently working out so well for some women whilst leaving a great dirty stain on the lives of others?

Jacqui had worked in a number of different clubs up north as a way to fund her university degree. But she, like Karen, had found that it wasn't the easy dollar she thought it would be.

'The thing about lap dancing — what you don't realise until you're finished with it and you're looking back — is that it's so *weird*. There are these men you've never met before in your life and they come in, give you some money, and you take your clothes off for them. It's bizarre. You have these conversations with people that you would never have in a normal situation — I remember this one guy who started going on about the size of my nipples, and I had to just carry on dancing and chatting to him. And when you're working in an environment which is that abnormal, it's very hard not to let it affect your life outside work.'

I asked Jacqui why girls like Sarah seemed to be having such a good time and making so much money if that was the case.

'When you're actually working as a dancer, you're not going to admit that you're not making loads of money. If you do, then you're basically admitting that you're not very good at your job — and part of the whole act is making out that you're desirable and every man wants to pay to spend time with you. And aside from all that, everyone has their pride. Who's going to admit that no one wants to see you take your clothes off?'

What seemed to bother Jacqui most was not the barely hidden layer of prostitution or even the less-than-enchanting customers. What bothered her, and what was increasingly bothering me, was the insincerity of it all — the women pretending to be interested in their customers, the managers pretending that girls were making a fortune in their clubs, the whole industry pretending that this was a normal Friday night out on the high street.

What also bothered me was the hypocritical dichotomy of it all. On the one hand lap dancing had become acceptable; men were now perfectly willing to admit that they visited lap dancing clubs, often with the apparent blessing of their wives and girlfriends. But the women I met who had worked in the clubs couldn't admit to their families or potential employees that they had worked as a dancer — let alone go on TV to talk about it. When I began looking into lap dancing I thought it was the men who were being taken for a ride. I thought that the women who were objecting to it were oversensitive busybodies, unable to accept that people could pay for a sexual experience or jealous that they did not have the body or the confidence to do it themselves. Talking to Jacqui had made everything fit into place. I had fallen into the trap of thinking that it wasn't my place to object to lap dancing because women were doing it by choice. It finally hit me how naive I had been, and just how heavily the industry relied upon the naivety of women like me.

Jacqui, like the others, did not want to appear on camera, but by this time I was determined that the dancers' stories should form a part of the film. I finally found someone who would be filmed – a pole dancing teacher who used to work in the clubs. She did her interview anonymously, but talked about the Darwinian nature of the clubs, the fact that women who wanted to make money had to be prepared to go that bit further to get the customers: the things that all the other women had spoken about.

But that was not the story the broadcaster wanted. As we edited the footage together and showed them various versions of the film, we were told that there needed to be more nudity at the beginning, more suggestion of the titillating footage that was to come. When the programme came out – all grainy footage and breathless commentary about the debauchery that could be bought on the high street – it felt as though it was a promotion for the clubs. I doubt whether any of the ones we featured lost any business because of it; in fact I am convinced that many of them would have seen an upturn in trade. Perversely the film had only added to the forbidden allure of the clubs – it had done little, if anything, to tell it from the dancers' perspectives. The interview with the pole dancing teacher was relegated to part three of the programme, almost an afterthought.

I had failed the women who had opened up to me. They had spoken to me, a stranger, about things they probably hadn't spoken with their own family about, but the programme turned out as little more than a salacious piece of soft porn. Soft porn with a faux judgemental voice, but soft porn nonetheless. It was another lie about lap dancing, another little piece of insincerity to pile on top of all the others. Our film was meant to expose lap dancing; instead all it did was portray the dancers as immoral tarts who were out to make as much money as possible. The people behind the whole industry escaped any kind of criticism.

The story still bothers me because I never managed to tell it properly. If I was being political about it I might claim that the programme turned out as it did because television commissioners are overwhelmingly male. In reality I know that it's because broadcasting, like lap dancing, is a market. To attract the advertising revenue you have to bring in the viewers, and viewers would rather see naked women than be lectured on the loopholes in the Licensing Act. So maybe that's why, a year after the programme was aired, I still feel the need to argue my point vociferously whenever I get into a conversation about lap dancing. When people say that lap dancers are raking it in, I have to contradict them. When they try to tell me that it's all just a bit of light-hearted fun, I can't let it go.

I don't think lap dancing should be banned, but I do think it needs to be laid open and shown for what it is. Women need to know exactly what they're getting into rather than being sold an illusion. Instead of being left to operate how they choose, the clubs should be forced to take all their dancers on as employees and pay them a set wage. And the licenses should be expensive enough and difficult enough to obtain to make sure than those who do get them don't allow activities on the premises which could see their licenses being revoked.

My opinion has changed. Lap dancing is a feminist issue, but not because of objectification. Women are constantly objectified whatever they do, as are men — that's not something a campaign is ever going to change. The real issue with lap dancing is more serious than that: it's about poor working conditions and false job descriptions and workplace intimidation. It's about an industry which relies entirely upon women, yet grants its female employees few if any rights; in that sense an industry that's stuck in the mindset of a pre-Equal Pay Act era.

As I began writing this I decided to get back in touch with Sarah. I wanted to find out if she had started university, whether she was still lap dancing, if she was still enjoying it. I wanted to see if she was still making the kind of money she claimed she was making when I met her, now that the recession had really taken hold. I wanted to know if she was still with her boyfriend, and whether he still brought his mates into the club to show her off. So I wrote all my questions in an email and sent it off to her.

I never received a reply.

Student

I was a student and heard from a friend that the topless bar in town had jobs going. She only mentioned it in passing. It was odd, because no one encouraged me to go or egged me on, but somehow I just felt curious about it. I went along and asked the manager for a job, and there was no audition or anything. I ended up working there for about nine months, as a 'dancer' (as we termed ourselves) as well as behind the bar.

I think I had a sense of topless dancing being a daring, edgy thing to do. That it was bold – not something people who knew me would expect. So it was more an egotistical choice than anything else; I didn't want for money, as I was very well supported by my family.

Where I worked was a fairly small place, just a small pub really, but with blacked out windows. It wasn't always warm enough, especially on evenings when there weren't many customers so you couldn't keep busy. All the women worked 'independently', meaning we were in direct competition with each other. We were working for ourselves and not the owner – or that's how he wanted us to see it at any rate. We each had to pay a fee for the privilege of working – £20 on quieter nights, £30 on Fridays and Saturdays. We didn't have to drink but it was definitely encouraged. The 'house' drink that customers were encouraged to buy us was a glass of 'champagne' at £5 each. We would take the money to the bar ourselves, but actually ask for a lemonade instead, and pocket the difference. This was seen as clever, enterprising – in an environment where everyone is seen as exploiting everyone else, what's wrong with lying about something like that? Exploitation was the norm.

In terms of the rules at the club at first I was quite naive. I remember dancing with a customer once, and one of the other women came over immediately and told me off – I didn't realise what I had done was against the rules. I'm still not sure what it was I actually did wrong. There was a point when things at the club changed and a number of dancers who were apparently from a large successful club arrived. They had a much slicker style, with Ann Summers-style out-fits, breast implants, pre-arranged routines, headstands, doing the splits – we looked like poor relations by compar-ison. I vividly remember one woman putting her finger into her vagina, drawing it out again and waving it under the customer's nose so he could smell it; this happened often, and a number of the women did it. They charged more for that. They also had an impossible-looking move that involved doing a headstand right in front of the customer and spreading their legs wide open. I heard that one woman did occasionally let customers put a finger in her vagina, but I don't remember seeing that.

The effect of this was that there was an expectation from the customers that the rest of us would do the same things. Not that we were innocent and they were guilty – they were just much more full-on. That made me think that what they were doing must be the norm at those bigger successful clubs – you don't all learn to dance in the same way unless it's taught or shown to you. We didn't get shown what to do, so our styles differed more. They seemed like they'd come off a production line.

Why did I eventually leave? With hindsight it's easy to say it was because deep down I knew it wasn't alright – but I honestly didn't analyse it much at the time. There wasn't anyone I could talk to on a level about it, because my friends were by definition outsiders. So I didn't have in-depth conversations about it. I just started to find it more and more of a chore, less and less fun, and I got ripped off once by the manager, which I think added up to a desire to give it up.

Some people say it is easy money, sometimes it felt very easy – on busy nights. I remember one man would slip me a fiver every few minutes, winking, saying it was for the tuition fees. I'd smile and laugh along. That was easy. But really, on a slow night I sometimes earned less than I would have done in a shop or a normal bar.

A couple of the other women were involved in prostitution, but conversations about our lives outside the club were pretty rare, so I don't know exactly what that involved for them. I asked one of them if it was possible to work as an escort but not have sex with the clients, and her response was, '… ain't nothing wrong with a little sex, girl'. She made it sound like she was fairly in control, and like she'd been doing it for a long time. In terms of the customers, I don't recall being propositioned or expected to be available for sex, but I think the opportunity was certainly there if I'd sought it out.

I don't think that topless dancing is empowering for women – it is empowering for men. And it's not just sexual – these men like being in an environment where women give them lavish attention, laugh at their jokes, flirt with them and ultimately get their tits out for them. Women in the 'normal' world are not usually so biddable. The difficulty is that it feels empowering, because you feel that you have something the man wants. I think most of us don't take the trouble to distinguish between whether this power is real or just a feeling, an illusion. And let's face it – if you're a woman working in the lap dancing industry, for whatever reason, it's a hell of a lot more comfortable to believe that you're empowered than to believe you're deluding yourself. As Mary Wollstonecraft put it so distinctly in 1792: 'The illegitimate power which [women] obtain by degrading themselves is a curse.'

I think some women do get something out of it. I knew a lovely woman who worked at the club, who told me that she had mentioned her interest in lap dancing to her brother, who had told her she'd be no good at it. She was proud of herself that she made decent money doing it and had proved she was good at something. Another woman said she'd never been good at anything before, and the improvement in her confidence and, actually, happiness, was easy to see. I can't begrudge those women the value that lap dancing had in their lives; many of us don't get any validation or encouragement from anyone. We're vulnerable to the messages of patriarchy because it's easier to get a job taking your clothes off than to build a life built on self respect. Self respect is really difficult to achieve for most of us, and we need help to do it. We don't need help to be lap dancers.

There are many reasons why we don't take issue with the industry: we don't know how to or even that we can; our good old British reserve; we think that women only do it willingly, and it's up to them what they do. Men sneer at us when we express doubt or disdain for the sex industry. Men still have an incredible power over women, and we're flattered that they want to pay to see our bodies. We've been taught to be this way. They're teaching our kids to be this way.

Bella

My life as a professional dancer — where do I start? Dancing has played a massive part in my life, both positive and negative. I first started out as a podium dancer at the age of 16 and had dreams of being a backing dancer in pop videos or in concerts. I had a diploma in performing arts, and performing in all aspects was my dream. I left college hoping and applying to get into university — not the average ones though, the best back then was LIPA (Liverpool Institute for Performing Arts). Unfortunately I didn't get in, as it was crazy. There were 500 people auditioning for 40 places, so it was really unlikely that I would get in anyway. I decided to take a year out and try again for the same ones rather than go for the ones I was offered, as I wanted the best. I continued to podium-dance every weekend in the top clubs in Manchester. I was admired for my talent and loved every minute of it.

Sadly I had a horrific life-changing experience. I was shot three times by four men who let off 36 rounds (the police told me after), so they meant to kill. I was in the wrong place at the completely wrong time. From this moment on my life changed dramatically. I started drinking, taking drugs and attempted suicide many times. On one occasion I died and was brought back to life. So you could say I was a mess, and it lasted a couple of years. As time went on I started to remember who I was and began building myself back up. I started dancing professionally again and became part of a group which broke up after a year, but my confidence was coming back. Then I met the women who changed everything. One of them was going out with my cousin and was a lap dancer who danced in Manchester. I looked down at this as I considered myself as a professional dancer, hired for my talent, but as it goes I really got on with her, and she introduced me to her world: footballers, parties and good times. After what I had been through, this seemed like an amazing, glamorous life, so after months of persuasion I finally gave in. Who wouldn't? I earned £35–£40 per night for 30 minute energetic, sweat-and-talent-packed sets, and she earned up to £500 a night. Oh my God, I couldn't believe it! So, she introduced me to her agent. Back then you had to have an agent to get in at any club. The agent thought I would be perfect, so I started.

My first night was at a fabulous club in the Midlands. It was run by a couple. There was a DJ who introduced us all one by one. We had to wear long classy dresses as we were high class ladies, weren't we? We started with 'elegance hours' with the long dresses, then we had 'fantasy hour', then any costume after midnight, as long as it was tasteful and sexy. When I walked in the room I was surrounded by glamorous, sexy, strong, independent ladies who all had Mercedes or BMWs parked outside, bought from their own cash. I was in, and couldn't believe it! I came from lying on the floor filled with bullets, waking up in a mental home after so many suicide attempts to being accepted into the same league as these women.

Anyway, I got my first dance. Back then it was £5 topless, £10 full nude. I was terrified, but here we go — I was introduced as Bella. I stood in front of a mature, wealthy looking man who smiled and was really lovely and warm and friendly. This was a doddle. I got in my zone; I was a professional dancer and had a show to put on, but a seductive type. I became fixed on his eyes and couldn't move as the nerves kicked in. I continued to look deep into his eyes, which became weird as it felt that there was no longer anyone else in the room. I suddenly became Bella, a strong, sexy, independent lady ready to seduce, and I loved it. I took control intensely. I leaned forward and put my hand on the bars behind his head, always conscious of the no-touching rule; I left space between us but could feel the tension. I slowly moved so my breasts were on eye level, still holding on to the bars I gave them a little shake. I looked down and he seemed to be in a daze — that feeling was great. I felt sexy and breathed with a sigh of relief. It aroused him even more as my breath touched his ear by accident. I then took my finger and lifted his chin up to look in my eyes; I suddenly became powerful and thrived on it. I then stood up and carried on with my sexy dance. As I turned around to do a grind move, I suddenly remembered where I was. Everyone was looking at me, the girls in shock as it was my first dance, men with their hands in the air beckoning me to do them next. It was amazing. I was Bella, and no one could tell me that what I was doing was wrong.

My cousin's girl was right, I was making silly money: £400,

£500 sometimes £600 a night. It was a blessing in disguise. My parents didn't like it but were glad I was out of the gutter I had accidentally fallen in. I went all over the country lap dancing. It was fabulous: going to VIP parties, doing footballers' private Christmas parties. I had clothes made for me. I got back into podium-dancing one night a week, went on amazing holidays, moved out of the council house, off 'the sick' and back to being independent, strong and happy again, and full of ambition. I soon became a stilt walker, going to different auditions for music videos, adverts, etc. My lap dancing was financing my rent, my clothes and costumes to get me to auditions. It was a great stepping stone for me, but slowly and surely things started changing.

As time went on, more and more clubs started opening, which meant more competition. I watched as the game stepped up and girls became bitchy and jealous, and all of a sudden it was dog-eat-dog. I was never worried because for me it was a stepping stone, as I had my podium dancing, stilts and all other jobs to fall back on, but some of these girls' lives depended on it. The pressure was on. More and more girls started working. Club fees went up and the tax man was getting on to the thousands that were lining young girls' pockets, tax free, for years. Not me though. I always declared mine through my accountant (honest!).

Throughout this change I remained the same and so did my dances, but others became competitive. What was once fun, glamorous and rewarding became dull, sleazy and degrading. I watched those strong independent ladies, whom

I looked up to once, slowly self-destruct. Don't get me wrong, some girls had their heads screwed on. Yes, I was one of them. I mean nothing lasts forever, so you always need a backup plan, or fingers in other pies.

One of the worst experiences was at a new club. I was out of my comfort zone, I didn't know anyone, and it was cliquey, but it had more money. In there, one girl had a millionaire who would always have dances with her. He bought her expensive things and she would see him outside of work. One night I made no money. I wouldn't change my dancing to the rude, sleazy stuff. In this club there was a private room and I know people had sex in there. I drank that night. I had made no money. I was pissed off. The millionaire's girl told me to come for some speed. I was not into that but I was in a strange, frivolous mood, and I had had enough of work, so I took it. It was white powder. That's the last thing I remember.

I woke up and someone was performing a sex act on me. I was hysterical. Girls were laughing. I was in a bedroom with this guy, the millionaire. I was screaming for help. Then another girl came in saying, *calm down*. I ran out, went home to my house. Telling my mate, we went to the police. When I thought of telling the police, I still saw myself as a professional dancer. I was in a bubble. When I talked to the police and described my job, I realised how sexual it was. The way they looked at me, I felt horrible. I kept trying to justify to them what I was doing. I wasn't asking for it — what happened in that bedroom. Just because I had taken drugs and take my clothes off for a living, I didn't have a leg to stand on.

This guy was a millionaire. The club backed him because he was one of the best customers. I never went back there. I was sacked anyway. I never saw the girl again; I carried on and blanked it out of my mind.

Eventually I stopped dancing as I was in a full, serious relationship. I became pregnant, but then the relationship failed while I was pregnant. I ate loads and became massive. After I gave birth I worked in retail. My body was no longer a way to make money; my self esteem was shattered. I was just a working mum. I had no relationships with men as I didn't feel sexy. After three years of this I woke up and thought how was I going to exercise, get money and meet people? Feel attractive again, like a woman. I thought, I am going back dancing: it builds your confidence, it's good exercise and you can socialise. I wanted the attention of men to boost my confidence. I still felt like an elephant. I started again in an old club with a new manager. I was a size 14. My boobs were massive. So the men didn't look at my belly, I wore a basque so that I never showed my stomach. It was horrible as all the girls were young and skinny. It was a battle to have the courage to leave the changing room, but I used my personality and my big boobs, that weren't fake, and was one of the top earners.

The new girls couldn't put on a show, they just stripped. There was no DJ, just CDs, and no elegance hour. It was not glamorous at all anymore. It was just a body in front of you, literally just sex: no glamour, no ambience, no atmosphere. It was stripped bare, just a woman naked, no showmanship. It did start feeling dirty. I just blocked it from my mind – that's why I did well. I could still perform, but that soon wore off. I worked in another club, but there you could grind, everyone was on coke, and it was so cliquey, but I knew some girls from the past. I watched girls grinding, rubbing themselves on the men, and putting their boobs in their face. I danced different, but soon it was not good enough.

I started drinking heavily again and grinding. It was horrible to feel someone's erection rubbing against you. I became like one of those girls drinking to get through the night. I couldn't justify what I was doing. I thought I needed the freedom and the money that it gave me, to live and aspire to be something more than I was. I was one of the girls I used to look down on. I did lose weight, and in some ways I did build my confidence up. The grinding became normal, and it wasn't as horrible. Throughout this I was aware of what I was doing and that it was wrong. I couldn't justify it. I had to stop to become a better person. But when do you stop, when the consequence is that the money stops? And how am I going to pay my bills and support my child? I started doing a project for youth. I was getting contacts from the lap dancing clubs to help with the youth club. I used the club for networking. I had contacts who were customers who became associates in my new venture.

I finally stopped dancing, It wasn't making me feel good. I had got what I needed, lost weight, made money. It had gone past the point of value; but I didn't really stop. I did fund-raising nights, 'gentleman's nights', because I knew the industry. I did it all nice, and put on a good night, but after I wondered, What am I doing? I was inviting family, friends and local people, but from their reaction I realised this was a bad thing. I was getting guys to come and pay to watch women take their clothes off. I saw it in a completely different light.

During both times I worked, I got different things out of it. First was getting the money. I had a nice body and had confidence. The second time it restored my confidence and made me feel sexy and like a woman again. But I was one of the lucky ones. Despite all the horrible things that happened, even what happened in that room, with that man, I feel fortunate.

When I left, I left a world with girls who had sex with customers in back rooms and dancing for hardly any money. It wasn't a show anymore. It was a meeting ground for prostitution. It didn't stop at dances. It shifted from this glamorous, eventful, fun world to a dark, shallow, horrible one; but I do have good memories, and I did well out of it. I would never change my experiences. It gave me skills for life and endless stories to tell, however I am pleased to say, *Goodbye Bella, it was nice knowing you.*

Prostitute

I worked in various brothels in and around London. I had previously worked in prostitution in Germany, having been pimped by my boyfriend. I mainly worked for one woman who, along with her husband, ran saunas/massage parlours.

There was a clear link between the lap dancing clubs and the brothels, although not formal. It is known that taxi drivers (including licensed black cabs) can receive commission for taking groups of men to lap dancing clubs. However there were also minicabs that would then pick up punters from the lap dancing clubs and bring them to the sauna. They would receive about £20 from the maid for bringing a group of men.

These punters could be some of the worst. There was a very aggressive 'pack mentality' and they would often be very rude and would be grabbing, slapping and touching us in the main seating area. They would often make very degrading comments about the way that women looked, often referring to women as 'mingers'. They invariably asked for group sex – it seemed important for them to have sex in front of their friends.

If they had been taking coke (which was quite often), or were too drunk and not able to get an erection or come in front of their friends, they would take it out on us for not doing our job properly or not turning them on enough, and would sometimes try to demand their money back. The sauna very rarely refused entrance to drunk or high punters, especially if there was a group of them, as it would mean losing out on too much money. Nor were we allowed to refuse them.

I think that the fact that the men had come from the lap dancing clubs meant that they had already stopped seeing us as human or individual. They would pick out women one after another to try out, to swap over, and to score in terms of 'performance'. The overwhelming feeling that I got was that they really hated us.

During a period in which I wasn't working, I was contacted by the brothel owner and she asked to meet up. She told me that she was planning to open up a lap dancing club. She had previously been prosecuted for running brothels so she was aware that it was risky to continue operating her saunas. She told me that she could see why I no longer wanted to work at the saunas because of the high number of foreign women there (most of whom I know for a fact were trafficked) and that I had 'moved beyond that'.

What she proposed was that me and a group of other women who were working for her become escorts. Through doing this we could start paying her money (on top of the usual cut she would take) to get a 5% share in the lap dancing club. Her proposal was that, once opened, the lap dancing club would act as a front for prostitution, and it was made very clear that the women would be expected to have sex with punters either on or off the premises.

I guess she saw this as a way of continuing her prostitution business but with less risk of the premises being raided. I declined her offer and I don't know whether she opened the club.

Waitress

I began waitressing at a strip club whilst at university. I know many girls who would get all dolled up, dance the night away on stage, take their knickers off in-between the knees of a customer, but go home in debt, due to the club charges. When asked why they would do this, especially as many of them had a successful day job, they would answer honestly that they enjoyed the attention. They relished the fact that they felt in absolute power when a man handed them money because he thought they were sexy. The fact that that very same money was being taken away from them by other men who ran the club did not make them realise they were not really the ones in power. They were not, in their eyes, being exploited or discriminated against.

Other girls were coerced into it by domineering and abusive partners, peer-pressured by groups of friends all doing the same thing and, saddening as it is, there were increasing numbers who were forced into it through abuse or slavery. Others were actually using it as a 'liberator' – those who had escaped sexual slavery, abusive and violent partners and saw their new occupation as the ultimate symbol of taking their freedom back, earning independently and becoming emotionally unavailable. The majority, however, would claim that they were intelligent women, there simply to make the most money they could in the shortest time possible in order to pursue what it was they really envisioned as their life's adventure.

I remember when I was a waitress in the club that we were not under as much pressure to lose weight/have a tan/make sure hair and make-up was perfect etc. as the performers were. However, waitresses were still given nightly 'inspections' by the (male) management to ensure the correct uniform (stockings, suspenders, corset, French knickers) was being worn in an appropriate style. The male waiters, however, who did EXACTLY the same job as the females, were required to wear trousers, a waistcoat and a bow-tie. They were generally never 'inspected' and enjoyed far more perks than any of the girls could hope to grab. The potential of promotion was very real for them, but something that was a distinct impossibility for the waitresses.

Managers and other staff treated the waitresses with slightly more respect than the performers in some aspects, but this was mainly due to the necessity of closer daily working interactions. Waitresses had a strict rota and were much more likely to be disciplined if they failed to show up for a shift or had a number of sick days. Performers were more in control of their schedules, and could usually swap nights more easily.

Waitresses were not encouraged to be too friendly with customers, just professionally flirtatious and smiley. If they wanted us to sit with them and talk, a manager had to be asked. If a customer did take a liking to a waitress, the performers would undoubtedly make complaints about her conduct, and react with school-girl claws. A waitress did not have to pay the club to work there. They received a paltry shift payment, a percentage of the service charge and their own tips, which differed greatly from the performers, who had over £100 per night in charges and up to 25% of their earnings taken by the club.

Waitresses were under a closer watch than performers in some ways. We could not stand around and chat, stay too long at a table, openly have a drink. The performers were paying to be there, so they had more freedom in the sense that they sat and laughed, sipping drinks and smoking (before the ban) – all part of the atmosphere creation. We were made to stand to attention with trays-at-the-ready at all times.

I remember for the performers the official rules were no touching at all, and a 'three-foot rule' – which meant all dancers were supposed to remain three foot away when performing. The three-foot rule was hardly ever adhered to, especially as lap dances really were 'lap' dances – hard to do that with three-feet in between! If the bouncers ever saw men touching the dancers, the customer would be reminded of the rule. If the actions were repeated, they often got thrown out. However, if it was a big spender in one of the VIP areas, the girls and bouncers would usually turn a well-paid blind eye.

Many of the dancers would go home with no money, even leaving work owing the club money, having not done enough dances to pay their fees. Some of the weekend workers, who had day jobs, seemed to make no money, bought their own drinks, and were doing it for the 'fun' and 'confidence boost', in their words. However, in my opinion these were a minority. The majority of the workers made a decent living from the job, sometimes having exceptional nights, pocketing a grand or so, but then experiencing other nights where cash flow could be as low as 50 quid. A few regularly made extravagant amounts – but this really did equate to 5–6% of the dancers, and there were always rumours about the 'extras' they offered to be recipients of such large payments.

Some people may think that I am a hypocrite for speaking out about an industry I made money in, but bankers are currently speaking out about the fundamental wrongs of their system, even though it is this system that has made them millions. It may seem hypocritical, but at the time you are just another person looking to make a living, and any reservations you have can seem secondary. It is only when you have had the experience that you can come to realisations and conclusions about the system you have worked in, and try to alert others to both the positives and negatives as honestly as possible.

Due to the fact that I made the money to pay my way through an expensive undergraduate and postgraduate university education from the industry, I cannot be vehemently against it. I am unsure whether, as a young girl with no other forms of financial assistance, I would have had the wherewithal to make that kind of money elsewhere. Chances are, my education certainly wouldn't have advanced as far as it did. However, in retrospect it angers me that, as an 18-year-old girl, I did see the industry as offering the most lucrative rewards with the minimum amount of time and effort required. In actual fact, it resulted in a complete lack of social life/friendships/activities etc. at university, and many close calls with expulsion due to missing more morning classes than even the most lively night-lovers in my year.

It also brought along its own huge bag of issues, that eating baked beans in a shared student house for five years might not have. What I wish to challenge is the normalisation of this as an obvious career choice for young girls, who are momentarily stuck for cash or in search of a quick financial fix. It is not easy money in the long run. There are definitely prices to pay — even if they're not monetary.

Every dancer I met believed at that time that what they were doing was empowering. For some, I can't deny that it must have been. There were those who were escaping abusive relationships, etc. who had finally found financial freedom and a confidence to live independently — even if it was perhaps not the best environment for them long-term. There were those from countries where they would have been expected to marry and have sexual relations with men they didn't like, or choose. So, to be making their own money from men, without having to marry or even touch them, certainly felt empowering. There were also many under-privileged young women who had dropped out of school very early, some being almost illiterate. If they had not been dancing, they admitted they would likely be on the dole, with a baby or two. To them, the financial independence and illusion of glamour was a life-saver.

In all of these cases, I often felt that there was some sense of empowerment, as these particular women were so sure and confident about their choice. Those who had definite plans and had began to put them into action with their earnings – property development, private school for their children etc. – also made the line blurry for me, because they held such conviction about their lifestyle and career choice.

Those who seemed less sure about what they were doing always highlighted the case against empowerment: those whom you found crying in the toilets after men had refused to pay, or ridiculed them, or called them fat; those who, night after night, went home with almost nothing in their purses; those who had reached their early 40s and knew they couldn't continue much longer, but felt utterly powerless to do anything else; those who had nothing to show for their years of stripping other than Gucci handbags and a coke habit; those who were unable to have relationships, friendships, any sense of normality; those who let men touch them even though they squirmed, who accepted their sloppy kisses and arse-slaps for 20 quid, feeling sick inside; those who thought they'd only be there for a year, but found themselves telling that story 15 years and an equal number of failed relationships later.

After a few years of watching and learning, I decided that the men have always got the power. They run the industry, they hire the dancers, they stock the bars, they produce the currency, they choose who dances for them, they decide who goes home happy, they pay. And, as lovely as it may be to think that you are making them pay – that they are paying for the pleasure of your company – the only reason anyone is there at all is because the men are the ones with the money – and therefore, ultimately, the power.

I know some performers will disagree with what I have said here. On the one hand, I think there are many performers who see the business as being genuinely positive, e.g. empowerment, finances, etc. On the other hand, I think many of the performers exaggerate their opinions to help justify their choice to themselves. As this is something that constantly goes on between performers – a sort of mutual appreciation and encouragement for having found themselves in the business (which is a necessity for morale and strength, which speaks volumes in itself) – it is easy for some people to gloss over any reservations or negative opinions they may hold. I do believe it is only possible to have a really clear, independent opinion on it when you have actually left the industry. If performers were performing whilst consciously agreeing with arguments against the industry, it would make life very difficult for them mentally, so I think many of them block it out until they know they are close to leaving.

The men who visited the club where not all the same – different attitudes were encountered every day. Some were the epitome of respect, and appreciated intelligence and wit, entertaining many girls with their own stories and humour. Some never had naked girls around them, but would come to chat without being viewed as a prowling pervert in a normal bar or club. Some were absolutely rude and disgraceful, constantly being warned or thrown out for touching/grabbing/not paying.

There were men who held the attitude that they should never have to pay for a woman. There were those that only ever wanted a woman they'd paid for, and those that believed the women really fancied them. There were embarrassed and polite men, who had come for a group party and told everyone about their wife, and confident and leery men who had four girls dance at a time. With a few major exceptions, generally there was an attitude of carefully drink-hidden disdain, begrudgingly mixed with absolute awe.

Everyone is different. But to explain the main attitude above – 'drink-hidden disdain, begrudgingly mixed with absolute awe' – I would say that they subconsciously or consciously resented the fact that these women wouldn't be talking to them if they weren't paying. That made them feel small and inferior. However, the women were often so outwardly confident, sexy and sometimes absolutely stunning, that a natural awe would occur, as the men would want them to fall at least a little in love with them, if only for the night.

I think that despite all the negatives I have highlighted, women still want to be part of this industry. There is an exponential increase in the sexualisation of society in general, and the objectification of women. This has made it an industry that has grown and become acceptable as a place of work: desirable to be seen as being desirable. If you are getting paid for how you look, this is close to being a celebrity –

which many would see as a good thing, in this celebrity-obsessed age. The stories of fortunes made and millionaires married are ubiquitous, and, when money rules, become a kind of 'career choice'. I think the main reasons young women aspire to be in the industry is to have their desirability verified by a fawning, paying, male audience, and to take the opportunity to make what is often seen as 'easy money' without having to train/study etc.

People often criticise burlesque, but I enjoy burlesque. Although it has no doubt helped in the normalisation of strip clubs, it shouldn't be regarded as the same at all. The burlesque shows are humorous. To me, they are laughing at the desire of both sexes to see flesh. It never appears very sexual to me, more of an artistic outlet for dressing up and being silly. It really is a skill, as the comedy performance must be present, or they wouldn't be successful. It is completely different to hustling for money from men who want your breasts in their face.

However, I feel completely different about pole dancing exercise classes. This I'm much more negative about. I think it's terrible that a young girl can accompany her mother to the gym and see pole dancing lesson posters. That a young boy will grow up thinking that's a normal thing for girls to want to do, and with the underlying knowledge that could bring, i.e. that they are at the gym to look good for him. I think it has done so much to make people view stripping as a 'fun' way to make a living, which is a huge U-turn for women in this day and age – that keeping fit is all about keeping sexy.

So what was the final turning point that led me to leave? Well, I left waitressing because I couldn't face putting on the awfully revealing uniform anymore, when half my colleagues were fully-covered, tuxedo-wearing men. I couldn't face the strict rules which had incongruously been put in place at a location where the most ridiculous things happen every night. I hated that I had no social life and lost contact with all my friends and the real world. I hated that I started to hate men and think that all men went to strip clubs and acted like the idiots we saw on a nightly basis. I'm so glad I left and realised how warped that vision is, how many lovely men there are in the world, and how much more there is to life than making money.

It made me grow up quicker than I would have liked. It made me wary of most men, quick to judge them and slow to trust. It made me have a very negative sexual image for a long time. It made sex seem unconnected with anything that could be loving and safe. It made me devalue myself as to what I could do outside of the industry. I felt tainted with its brush, and felt that there was so much hypocrisy. Stripping is so ubiquitous and apparently acceptable, but people still couldn't accept you for serious work if you said you'd been a stripper, or even just worked as I did in a strip club.

I felt I'd failed myself in terms of ambitions for my life, my work, my career. It made me realise how far women were from being equal, and it made me so very angry. In terms of new women entering this industry, I acknowledge that everybody is different and it's hard to advise against something you have done yourself without sounding hypocritical. But I would still say, *Don't*. There are so many other things you can do. Look into every single one of them before you think of lap dancing. If you have a single doubt, follow that doubt and let it lead you to your dream another way.

Wife

A couple of years ago, my then fiancé was to attend a stag weekend event for his closest friend. My fiancé was to be best man at his friend's wedding and therefore had a fairly major part to play.

My fiancé advised me that his friend wished to go to a lap dancing club during one of the stag weekend's evenings, and although it was not his sort of thing, he felt he had to go along with how his friend wished to celebrate his stag party; especially as he was best man. I did not put up any argument about this, and at the time had actually never once encountered (in my then 28 years of life) the issue of strippers/dancers where it actually affected me, my life, my relationships, or anybody close to me.

Upon my fiancé's return from his friend's stag weekend, I discovered that the entire group had put money in 'the kitty' in order to pay for a lap dance for the groom, and also him as the best man. He apparently had no choice but to sit through a lap dance. I discovered this dance took place in a private room, separate from where the rest of their party were sitting/drinking. The groom had one lap dance on a stage for all to see, then a private one of his own. My fiancé felt that the other members of their stag party were not getting into the spirit of the event, so opted to pay out of his own pocket for a lap dance in order to encourage the others to join in the spirit of the event (again, this took place in a private room). I do not believe that this action encouraged any additional interest from the other members of the party. My fiancé also insisted that he felt pressurized to buy a dance because the girls were quite 'full on', and even after buying them a drink they would not go away – so buying a dance would rid him of the pressure.

This was the first I had heard that lap dances took place in private rooms. I am not sure why, and I am not saying it is any better or worse, but the fact they had lap dances taking place in private rooms really disturbed me. For some reason, I thought they were performed where the man was sat drinking, with his friends around him, etc. (I have also discovered that most of my female friends, relatives and acquaintances thought the same and, upon discovering the private room issue, were taken aback.) Perhaps this thinking is more along the lines of a table dance? I am not altogether sure.

I am sickened at the thought of putting any female through either dance performance type, be it a more public dance or a private dance. Neither seems a good option; but at that time, when the world of lap dancing was all new to me, I felt that the private room made it much worse. I do actually view a lap dance as a sexual experience, so in my humble opinion it breaches the relationship rules of fidelity. The men do not buy lap dances for anything other than visual, sexual stimulation. If they were buying the dance for the sake of seeing a dance, nudity or partial nudity would not be ultimately necessary! Conversely, the women only sell lap dances for visual, sexual stimulation; if they were indeed selling a dance for the sake of performing a dance, again, nudity or partial nudity would not be ultimately necessary!

Following on from the stag weekend, I continued to assess the lap dancing issue in my own mind and it upset me greatly. It really made me fall apart, and I was not altogether sure why. I had lots of things buzzing around my head. Treating a woman like a piece of performing meat. Men, that have this disposable income to throw about in such a gross fashion, feeling they can impose their buying power in this way. Allowing a female to demean herself fully naked in view of a man, yet she would go about her normal day in full clothing. Likening a dancer to a female relative, such as having a daughter who might become one, or a sister. Or, if your mother might have been one, and how my fiancé, or any man, would feel about this.

My fiancé was witness to my upset and the thoughts I was processing and tried to justify himself, as described above. He apologised for his behaviour and insisted that in all his 37 years, he had only been to a strip club once (again on a stag party), and actually walked out because the females looked so bored and the club seemed very run down. Although I was sickened with his behaviour (and his friend's, and all men that visit such establishments), I could see that he felt the peer pressure to join in, etc. Furthermore, I did not state my case, as it were, prior to him going, even though I was well aware they were planning to visit a lap dancing club.

I had to accept the situation and move on; however, I

impressed upon my fiancé that if he wished to have lap dances in future, or attend strip clubs and the like, he should continue in life without me, as I do not have any respect for such behaviour, and I would rather he left me out of his life if that was the manner in which he wished to conduct himself. I should not say I would have been happy for him to conduct himself in such ways by frequenting such establishments as lap dancing/strip clubs, but that I respect he is an adult and that he should do as he considers fair. If he rightly considers that type of behaviour to be fair, then let him get on with it, but not with me by his side. He insisted he did not feel comfortable in such places and would not go again.

Prior to our wedding my fiancé organised his own stag weekend abroad. The friend to whom my fiancé was best man was asked to be our best man, although he had no dealings with the organisation of the stag weekend, nor much part to play in the wedding as it was much smaller and more low-key than his own.

My fiancé assured me before he left that he would not be visiting/taking part in any lap dance/strip clubs, or the like. He advised me that one of his other good friends, together with his own brother, were notified that should there be any whisperings of setting-up such a visit, they were to put an end to it. I happened to see his friend the night before they were to leave. We were having a very typical, general conversation, and for some reason he blurted out to me that they would not be visiting any lap dancing/strip clubs. I was not expecting this to come into the conversation at all and was rather taken aback, as I had not made any such mention to him during our conversation. I had my fiancé's word and I trusted him.

When he returned I asked how it all went, where they went, how was the food, the city, the race-driving event he had planned, etc. He responded and spoke generally about the trip and how his friends had gotten on together, as there were several friends from different groups, such as friends he had grown up with but have now moved further afield, local friends he presently socialises with on a fairly frequent basis, friends from university, friends from football, etc. – all of whom only have one thing in common, and that is their friendship with him, but not necessarily with one another. The point being, it may have been difficult for all to get along well for an entire weekend, and as they did not know each other well, group thinking might be harder, with one or the other struggling to control any particular outcome. As it happens, the best man took the reins...

Two weeks or so after their return from the stag party, I happened to ask, quite out of nowhere and for no particular reason, as I was sincerely expecting the answer to be 'no': 'So, did you visit any girly bars?' He admitted that they had. I understood why he did not tell me immediately upon his return – so I did not labour the point, although of course, my trust was entirely broken.

My fiancé told me that he had a lap dance, in a private room, paid for courtesy of the other members of his stag party. One of the other members also had a lap dance; I believe this friend had two dances, actually, and that once my fiancé had had his, he waited for his friend's dances to finish, and then he insisted the group drink up and leave. Apparently, the waitresses were all topless, so some of the members of the stag party did not feel the need to pay for a private dance as they were more than happy with the view from the bar, so to speak.

My fiancé insists he was more of less hurdled out of a cab, directly into this lap dancing club and put in line, strong-armed by his friends. He had no time to think or act, and was far too drunk to make his own feet/legs or brain work. (I am not being sarcastic, he actually said as much.) He also said that he could not remember what the girl even looked like; what colour hair she had, nothing. THIS APPALLED ME. What kind of respect can a man have for a fellow human being, to allow her to demean herself in such a way, that he cannot even remember what she looks like? This female is somebody's daughter, possibly sister, mother, partner – and she dances naked for men so drunk and pathetic they do not have respect enough to acknowledge her as a fellow human being and recognise her physicality, her worth, her feelings.

I thought I just needed time to forgive him for this, but did not know how long it might take. We had the wedding fast approaching; our respective parents had given us a large sum of money to put towards the wedding and for our future home, etc. Wedding-related things had been booked, deposits paid, etc. Invitations had been sent, and I could not let everybody down by cancelling. After all, I was sure I just needed time to forgive him. As it happens, it took almost a year. This was after couples-counselling, and the idea to move out from our shared flat, to actually forgive him and have an understanding for how he had allowed this to happen.

But to this day, I still cannot forget that he did actually allow it to happen, and this is what haunts out marriage still. In truth, I have no regrets about how I have lived my life, perhaps what mistakes I have made, etc., as they are what have shaped me today. However, I do regret going through with the wedding. It was not the right time; I was thoroughly let down by the man I loved and respected. He showed no respect for me, our relationship, nor humankind. From this, I do not know yet how we are to move on.

I myself had a hen party prior to our wedding. My friends offered to organise it as I had enough on my plate with wedding preparations, and was thoroughly tired of it (weddings are not my thing, I am not a girly-girl and would have been only too happy to celebrate a quiet wedding, but I compromised, happily, for the sake of my loved ones and got on with it). My friends wanted to plan a surprise in terms of the content of the hen party, to which I agreed. I was asked what I thought about having a male stripper (this was after I found out about my fiancé's lap dance).

I said, quite honestly, that it was difficult for me to justify my reasons for disliking my fiancé's behaviour and to have an automatic opinion on the issue, as it had never entered my life before, nor had I any direct experience with lap dancing/ stripping. I therefore left it open to my friends' interpretations and gave them free rein. I was thoroughly confused, and I will say, not a single friend/relative/acquaintance of mine agreed with my stance against my fiancé's behaviour. I have therefore felt very alone in my thinking.

At my hen party, therefore, I had a stripper. He made me sit beneath him and forced my hands to rub his chest and legs (over his fake fireman's outfit). When he got up from me, to start taking off his fake fireman's jacket, I took the opportunity to stand up. He quickly turned and told me I had to stay seated, in a very firm manner. I apologised, saying this was not 'my thing', and made my exit to the garden beyond the patio doors.

A few friends came out from time to time to check I was OK. I was absolutely fine; it seemed the other members of my hen party were enjoying it, so although I felt terrible that they had wasted their money on me, at least they were making use of it (his services). My sister, apparently, took my place only too happily. So, not a complete waste. I think she enjoyed being the centre of attention. One friend of mine really tried to strong-arm me into returning to the party, but I insisted I would wait until the stripper was finished.

She later said I should lighten-up and it was all a bit of fun. I disagreed then and disagree now. I do not think she understood then, nor would she now; she is about 20 years my senior, and I suppose she has made her mind up in terms of morals and principles, and considers herself a mentor to me (she is an old family friend, who has seen me grow up). I am not ready to tackle her or many of my friends who view the issue as a bit of fun; I am simply not the type to do so, unfortunately.

I will copy below e-mail correspondence between my fiancé and myself, after one of our many discussions:

From: xxx@googlemail.com
Date: xx/xx/xxxx
Subject: can't do this by e-mail . . .
To: xxx@btinternet.com

My intention is not to hurt you. I feel completely lost. Am I your wife? . . . although my offer to become your wife was offered wonderfully, appreciated dearly and my feet didn't touch the ground for about fifteen months or so . . . when it came down to it, I felt the marriage vows were bestowed without grace, without sincerity. How could they be otherwise? You let me down monumentally. Over something which could have SO easily been avoided. I have been in despair ever since. My world came crashing down around me; the bottom fell out my world. All I can do at the moment, is to regain my own identity. I have NO intentions of hurting you, or trying to hurt you, but at the moment, I am not ready for you to have control of my heart again. I cannot allow myself to be put in that situation at the moment. I feel desperately alone.

From: xxx@btinternet.com
Date: xx/xx/xxxx
Subject: can't do this by e-mail . . .
To: xxx@googlemail.com

Hi Baby,

You are right we can't do this by email but I'll respond anyway.

I know I have hurt you enormously and it makes me feel physically sick every time I think about it. I know I have let you down and feel terrible that I was not able to honour a promise to you but I do

NOT consider that I've been unfaithful to you. I think this is where we have a fundamental difference of opinion. There was minimal physical contact but much more importantly to my thinking there was absolutely no emotional contact with this girl. I did not lust after her and I cannot even remember what she looked like. It is not an experience I took any enjoyment from at the time or since then. I have said this to you before but I need to repeat it. I had never been to a lap dancing bar before the stag weekend and never wanted to visit one again. This is not a situation that will repeat itself.

You asked the other day why on a recent stag weekend we didn't visit any lap dancing bars. I think the reason for this was two-fold, I was naive in thinking that we could avoid the seedier side of where my stag night was. With hindsight I should have avoided the place but I had already been on stag weekends in other countries where we had avoided such establishments, I thought we could here. The other reason was no one wanted to visit such places on these trips. The one person who I hadn't been on a stag weekend with was my best man. His view of stag weekends and the 'customs' of them had been formed from going on similar trips with fellow marines where a much more 'macho' culture prevailed. Whatever you, or indeed I, think of it, the visiting of lap dancing bars or strippers is very much a part of the culture of the armed forces. I suppose it is seen as a method of male bonding. Hence expressions such as 'Work hard play hard'. Soldiers and marines are trained to totally trust and support their comrades and not to think too much as individuals. If they did they wouldn't be able to kill people or, if they thought about the con- sequences for their families, they wouldn't be able to put them- selves in danger. This may seem like a very antiquated viewpoint but it still exists in my friend's world and he mistakenly thought that this is what I and the rest of the group wanted.

I know all the above does not absolve me of blame for what happened, but I am just trying to put it in context. I am guilty of poor judgement, being weak and most importantly putting my feelings of pride/shyness/insecurities before my commitment to you.

I totally stand by the vows I made at our wedding and it hurts deeply that you feel I was not being sincere. No matter how you feel, to me you are my wife. The saddest part of this is I think I know you better than anyone else in the world and you are unable/can't let me help or comfort you when you need me the most. (It's a good job everyone else has gone out because I am crying writing this.)

I know you are not deliberately or maliciously trying to hurt me but that is the side effect of your actions. I too feel desperately alone. I am constantly fluctuating between fear, despair, repulsion for my own actions, anger and I don't know what. We need to get through this . . . how I don't know . . . but at least in the meantime can we be alone together?

All my love,

xx

P.S. This was a lot longer than I originally planned!

*   *   *

I will copy below e-mail correspondence between a male friend and myself, following a discussion in relation to this subject:

From: xxx@googlemail.com
Date: xx/xx/xxxx
Subject: WARNING — ITS A LOOOOONG STORY, SO READ WHEN YOU HAVE TIME . . .
To: xxx@xxx.org

Thanks for asking about me. As I said before, living in the present is fine.

I will tell you the story, as I have a few spare minutes, as when we're all out together for dinner/drinks, it's just not really a good topic of conversation and will invariably send me off on an emotional rollercoaster.

My husband was fully aware of how I felt about strip clubs/lap dancing clubs, etc. He was apparently on the same page and promised his stag do would not involve visiting one. It did. He didn't tell me, I found out by asking in casual conversation several weeks later. I was shocked, as I was not expecting a 'yes' response and am not even sure why I asked, as I trusted him completely. I did not make him promise anything, he did it of his own volition. I tolerate such things going on, but out of choice would not choose a life partner who is not in opposition to this. It contravenes harmony in the relationship if you're not on the same page about moral issues. Obviously, you can't agree about everything, but when an issue is really important to the one you supposedly love, well . . . need I say more.

I stupidly went ahead with the wedding (having only found out two weeks prior), thinking that in time I could forgive him. It was too late to cancel after invitations had been sent, deposits paid, etc. . . . and although it has taken close to one year to forgive him, or at the very least, understand what went on, etc., I will never be able to look back on that summer as what was supposed to be a happy time. A special time, one to supposedly cherish forever. No. I do not feel married at all . . . and I didn't even care about the stupid events of the day . . . a small ceremony between just the two of us was all I needed. No effing white dress, fancy car, walking down the aisle — that's all girly rubbish. I'm not materialistic and was only hoping to have feelings of love on our wedding day.

The day was his, and his Mum's, and my parents . . . I actually feel like the typical bloke in the situation, as all I did was show-up, say a few words, my bit was done.

And the events of his stag do further proved that the marriage was his, as 'we' did not even feature as the reason behind it...

My opinion of the individuals who visit such establishments is that they do not value or respect women as fellow human beings, also made of flesh, who have feelings ... I know you've been to a few, so you would not agree, but we're each allowed our opinions. To live in a free society is wonderful and I embrace it, but I would not ideally choose to share my life with somebody who behaves so wholly against me, in terms of morals and principles. It would be like finding out he was drug pusher or was harbouring racist intentions.

I didn't think I was asking too much from our wedding ... and so was not expecting to then be so especially let down, humiliated, made to feel completely insignificant. If I was stomping around making unreasonable, expensive, irrational demands, like the stereotypical bride, I would expect the slap in the face I got. I got the slap in face, rather undeservedly methinks.

So you see, my husband and I will probably never be 'better'.

From: xxx@xxx.org
Date: xx/xx/xxxx
Subject: WARNING — ITS A LOOOOONG STORY, SO READ WHEN YOU HAVE TIME...
To: xxx@googlemail.com

Few points taken from the story:

1/ did he go to the strip club in the UK?
2/ It is (almost) obligatory for a stag do to involve some sort of nakedness (of the female variety) — also, please do not under-estimate the amount of implicit peer pressure that may have been exerted (not saying that he could not have resisted but...)
3/ Which upset you more, that he went or that he didn't tell you??

Yes, I have been to a few strip clubs, in the UK & when I have been on friends stag dos. I had a little night out with friends a few days before the wedding which included a strip club, so suppose my thoughts on these things are different (Dad came along as well, VERY FUNNY!!!).

For me, it is simply a little bit of titillation and nothing more than a little entertainment. You can see but not touch so it is 'frustrating', and once we went and we sat round drinking and chatting about our respective football teams (suppose you could say typical blokes!), the poor girls never really got a look-in. Actually in terms of 'exploitation', at a strip bar the general feeling is that you, the blokes, are being exploited, and it is the women that have the choice, the power and the control over us, plus they simply view it as a job and often look quite bored.

Also, I have always been totally honest with my partner about these things and have normally let her know these things in advance as well as informing her afterwards how the evening was. She is not really bothered by this and accepts it for what it is, but can see from your point of view that it is a big grey area and that you are not happy with any of it — I also know of two other friends wives who went through similar process and spent days crying, months to 'forgive' etc. so don't think your point of view is too unusual.

But, if she did have strong views on this then would I not go . . . or would it encourage me simply to lie about it . . . not sure really. Understand what you mean about being similar in terms of moral issues, me & my partner are similar it's just that these are different from yours.

OK yes, understand that you will never really be 'better' but personally think you should just make your feelings very clear to him (which I feel you will have done!), ask him not to do it again and then move on, otherwise you will let it fester and think there are probably bigger problems/challenges in life than this. Maybe a little perspective about what he did.

From: xxx@googlemail.com
Date: xx/xx/xxxx
Subject: answers to your questions . . . (another long-eeeeee)
To: xxx@xxx.org

Morning!

Hope you had a good weekend . . . Answers to your questions:

1/ Lap dancing club was abroad. Complete nakedness and touching allowed. This point does not bother me. I think it's extremely frustrating to be 'titillated' and for it to come to no fruition. He lost out — should have gone for the 'happy ending'; I would not have been in any way more or less hurt/disappointed. A sexual experience is a sexual experience. He says he doesn't remember what the girl looked like, what colour hair, etc. This is appalling. That girl is somebody's daughter, possibly somebody's sister or mother; she has degraded herself for a pathetic, drunken, middle-class sap; pranced around naked and he doesn't have the decency or respect to even remember what she looks like. I find this inexcusable, deplorable behaviour. Human nature is so unkind.

2/ The 'obligatory' bit smacks of lack of imagination, following the crowd. I thought my husband had own mind and did not follow convention for convention sake. Besides, he 'assured' me it would not happen. Do I or our relationship matter?

3/ Which upset me more? That he went. I understand why he did not tell me. Don't take this as any form of personal attack. My opinion is that the industry is soul destroying and I do not wish to be associated with such things. I feel a responsibility to fellow human beings to not allow them to undergo such harm. They look 'bored'. Why? Soul destroying. Is it healthy to work in such an industry? Is there room for promotion? Or, simply, 'demotion' into prostitution and further. Clubs which advertise 'new girls each week' (of which there are several) = human trafficking. It is irresponsible for me to support this industry, even in the remote way that I have, by staying with my husband.

Yes, there is a demand for the industry; there is also a demand for drugs therefore drug dealers exist and drug barons — destroying local economies in developing countries. Is this also OK, because there is a demand? It would be irresponsible for me to buy drugs. I recycle, give blood, etc . . . all in the name of human responsibility to society and our world.

If the blokes are apparently being 'exploited', why do it? Common complaint is that girls are only after blokes for their money. Is this playing right into their hands then? Self-fulfilling prophecy.

I am glad that all enjoyed the wedding. I made the compromise for the fairly 'big' event and was happy to do so . . . but even the very next day, we were discussing renewing our vows, as he knew full well he had let me and our relationship down. Similar to your wife, I wanted to feel like a princess too. Perhaps not in such an ostentatious manner, but my husband's princess, nonetheless. And don't laugh — I'm no princess to look at, I know, but you know what I mean. . . . You know something, a week before the wedding I went out with you guys . . . and you guys made me feel like a princess.

I do not look at the photos with fondness. Have not even had the album developed, which was paid for in advance . . . Thanks for the disc you copied and to all the other peeps whom did the same. Filed them away in the wedding folder, never once seen.

We have been to Relate and I fully understand why/how it happened, so I don't need any more perspective. My husband also fully understands my point of view and counsellor was able to relay my point of view to him without me even having to elaborate on the above, as I have with you and ALL of my friends.

I do however need to feel married and want to have an occasion to mark. Our official first anniversary is coming up . . . we'll be abroad and it will go unnoticed.

So, not sure how the future will pan out . . . but just taking every day as it comes.

I hope I haven't bored you silly and I implore that you do not take any of the above as any sort of personal attack. I value our friendship.

Hope to see you at the weekend then. . . .

Ciao-ciao xx

From: xxx@xxx.org
Date: xx/xx/xxxx
Subject: RE: answers to your questions . . . (another long-eeeeee)
To: xxx@googlemail.com

Heya

Actually agree with a number of your points!!!

1/ whilst touching allowed, I've not seen 'happy ending' available . . . Yes, also understand that being drunk and not having the decency to remember how they look etc., last lap dance I had spent about an hour chatting to the girl before hand (quite sad I know) but it was interesting as she was doing a Management degree so was giving her advice and felt a bit like a 'dad' actually. Yes, you should accept that they are people and have respect for them.
2/ aye, you are right here — plus it's been a while that I have been that drunk that I am not really responsible for my actions.
3/ hmmmm, never really thought about whether it leads women on to other things if they do not do well, fair point well made.
4/ are you against the whole 'sex' industry and where, for you, do you draw the line, pornography, 'lads mags' (Like *FHM*, *Loaded* etc.). Can see your point of view but just wondering where the line is in your opinion on what is acceptable and what ain't.
5/ yep, the blokes are being exploited, feel that the cleverer ones realize this and men go along with it.

And no, I don't take it as a personal attack, know that it is not intended in such a way and hope you feel that as a friend you can express your point of view without me taking it personally. I am easily able to accept an opposing view to mine without being upset.

Speak soon & don't feel the need to reply to my above points, as feel this discussion could go on and on and on... But we will always have different views.

Bya

P.S. — you ever been to a lap dancing club??

In summary, I have learned from this experience to question everything and to not adhere to convention for convention sake; to have an open mind about the consequences and effects of our actions, because through this we learn about responsibility to self and society as a whole, our community, our world — including all elements of nature and our environment.

Auditionee

A friend of mine mentioned that she wanted to audition for one of the biggest clubs in London, but wanted someone to go with. She knew I was quite confident about my body and asked me to come along. At first I thought it would be a fun experience. When she went to the audition, though, I had thought more about it and decided I would not be able to do it – more the pole dancing than the exposure bothered me then. She went and got it – she had worked in the Midlands as a stripper before drama school and was a great dancer.

A few weeks later I realised that I was totally broke. My parents and I were not on great terms at the time, and I decided that I couldn't pass up the chance to earn the kind of money my friend had mentioned. I went to the 'open auditions' at the same club my friend worked in, that were being held on Thursday evenings. As far as I know they still hold these.

I went to the back door and was let in and shown to the female toilets to change. My friend had told me to wear heels and an evening dress with just a thong. The idea, she said, was to go up onstage when they asked, take the dress off as fast as possible, and then dance around the pole for 30 seconds. There were four other girls there with me to audition. The club was not busy and there were no girls working, but the club was certainly not closed — people seemed to have gathered to watch the auditions.

The first girl I chatted to was very young looking — although she gave her age as 18. She was Polish and had come to this country on her own when she was a teenager. She said she came here to learn English and get some education. She had been working at a smaller club in London for two years on and off, but wanted to earn some better money. She asked me what my name was, and when I gave her my real name she said I should dance under a false name — something I was aware my friend had done. At that point another girl, very good looking and older than me (perhaps mid-20s), chipped in and agreed. She was quite aggressive and seemed to have worked as a lap dancer before too. She was sneering at me and my inexperience, and made it clear that she expected to get the job.

The other two there were both younger than me — perhaps just 18. One was quite thin and one was much chubbier, but neither could speak much English. By this point I was really uncomfortable, and I was grateful that the Polish girl was really chatty with me. She seemed as desperate as I was for money, so I confided in her that this was my last hope for this month's rent.

At that point a guy came over to us — sitting on sofas outside the ladies loo — and told us we would dance in two groups on the three poles on the main stage. It was a T-shaped platform in the centre of the room with three dancing poles. I went to the front pole and the Polish girl and the sneering woman took the back poles. The music came on and I took off my dress as fast as I could. I couldn't see the faces of the people in the audience, but I could hear the hum of them talking and laughing under the music. I tried to dance around the pole but did not do a good job, I suspect, as I was scared out of my mind! I just felt that I did not have the personal strength to be there. As soon as the music stopped we left the stage and dressed. I was shaking.

Then the other two girls danced. It was all over really fast and we all sat and waited for the men to come and tell us what they thought. It was really tense and I felt like throwing up. Part of me needed the job and hoped I had done enough, and part of me wanted to run away. Some other girls came in and chatted to the first man. They wanted to dance and the guy seemed to know them — he told one she didn't have to audition and she went through to the loo. He told the other one to come back next week.

Then he came to us and said we all needed to take some lessons in dancing on the pole, and we needed to tone up our bodies. Then he walked off and we went back to the changing rooms. I just wanted to leave and not speak to anyone, but the Polish girl asked me what I was going to do. I said I wouldn't come back. The sneering woman was really angry and left fast. The Polish girl offered to get me a job. At first I thought it was a chance to earn the cash I needed and considered it. She told me I wouldn't have to audition if I gave her name, and recommended I come and talk to her boss the next afternoon. We left and the bouncers led us out. One of them told us to come back in a few weeks. I felt worse then, seeing in the bouncers' eyes exactly how little they thought of us.

As we walked to the station together, the Polish girl explained about the job. She said I would be paid £50 to dance (different from the club I had just auditioned for where you pay £15 pounds at the start of your shift and £65 at the end). Then she described going around the bar with a pint mug before and after dancing. I was shocked. Then she told me about private lap dances which happened in a separate room. For that, she intimated that the price was agreed with the customer. She gave the impression that this involved bartering and I became aware that she offered 'extras'. At that point I went another way to her.

I was totally out of my depth here and I never went to the club she told me about. In fact, I threw away the contact details on the journey home. The whole experience was disgusting to me. I had seen my friend going and earning lots of cash – she seemed not bothered by the whole thing, I guess because she was used to it. Eventually, though, she gave it up – it was exhausting as she had to work certain shifts in the week and was fined if she could not make it. She said weekday shifts were not profitable and weekend shifts were very competitive. She described how women would pounce on any man who got out a credit card, and how the atmosphere was one of fear. Also, her partner at the time had a hard time dealing with it.

I had never thought about the effect of lap dancing clubs or the sex industry before this – always thinking these women had the power, etc. My one small encounter with that culture made me realise what foul places they really are, and I am ashamed of myself for being sucked into what I see as the 'sexual propaganda' which surrounds the industry.

Natasha

We are told about body confidence: look good naked, feel good naked, love your body, don't hide it, no shame in it, look at it, it's beautiful. This beauty can be shared; others can find it beautiful. No, better, others can find their beauty from looking at your body confidence.

I started work as a lap dancer after spending 10 years in a controlling relationship which had triggered a psychotic mental breakdown. Without going into too much detail, such episodes can certainly lower one's confidence! I finally had the courage to leave the relationship and do something that I wanted to do, regardless of others' views.

A little introduction: I'm a teacher, first and foremost. I teach English and Maths up to GCSE level. Everyone remembers me as a lap dancer though. Nobody ever asks me to write a piece about my teaching. I hope that this story will help demystify. The reality is I'm a lap-dancer and a teacher — there is no contradiction. Lap dancing is one part of my glorious identity, it maketh part of the woman, and I'm dammed if I feel forced to feel ashamed, apologise for it, or deny it in any way.

Anyway, I got to a situation with my ex which was just untenable for both of us, for many complex reasons. We split up but were still living in the same house. Around the same time I gave up my teaching job as I was struggling to maintain it because of my diabetes.

I went to London. On the way back, the coach was about to leave, the seat next to me empty. A young woman sprinted to the front of the bus, spoke briefly to the bus driver and plonked herself buoyantly beside me. She started chatting away. She was a lap dancer, said I should try it, but, well, the late nights and the constant consumption of alcohol were not the most healthy way to live...

Next time I went to London, it was for a singing audition. I had had some singing lessons and thought, *Why not?* Why not? Well, because my voice was untrained and I was uncommitted. One of the panel said, 'Why do you want to become a singer?' I mumbled something about using my voice. They were interested in my explanation, but not my voice! I don't blame them. Why do I want to become a singer? I don't really, I just want to do something in the realm of performance. What do I want to do – what have I always loved doing? Dancing! I get back on the coach and promise myself to go to the next dancing auditions in Birmingham. With no professional training, the lap dancing club I had been told about was the only option.

He kicked me out when I told him. (I thought he didn't care about me anymore, that's what he'd said the week before. He now told me I shouldn't have listened to him – I think he shouldn't have said he didn't care if he didn't mean it. During that conversation I gave him three opportunities to take it back, but he calmly told me three times that he didn't care. I listened to him – now I'm glad I listened, as there was a lot of truth in it.) I moved into a friend's house: a genuine friend who said that she would have lap danced if it wasn't for the stretch marks. Really, she should have done it anyway... What is it with women and their stretch marks? Perhaps I'll never understand. Body confidence — they are right, that's what we all really need.

She teaches me how to flirt, I really didn't know. Not something a PGCE teaches you — not something life teaches you if you have been raised through the Catholic convent education system — not that I'm knocking it at all. The part of me that is an inspiring teacher, that's partly due to that system. However there was no course in flirting. I needed that, now I understood it. I realised how it's just not me.

I went for three auditions at that club. I was told that I'll just never cut it. So I auditioned elsewhere. I got a job, learned how to pole dance, learned how to lap dance, never earned much money, but enjoyed the body confidence, the constant dancing, and my genuine friendships with the girls.

The girls! What amazing young women. These girls are businesswomen. They plan from beginning to end. They earn the money most of the time, they go home and live. Any person who depicts the lap dancer as a powerless woman does not know what they are talking about. They just don't have a clue. Yes, women are oppressed. When I walk into school and see that 90% of the staff are women but 90% of the management are men, I recognise that women are oppressed. When I see the disproportionate statistics of uneducated women across the globe, I know women are oppressed. I'm a black, bisexual young woman with an unseen, inadequately-treated disability. Honestly, I have some understanding of oppression, of societal oppression, of people not being able to quite treat you as a whole human being; of people just not being able to understand. I know oppression. Honestly. Using lap dancing clubs as any type of scapegoat for that oppression is just not helpful. It just doesn't help.

It denies the existence of educated women who make the conscious choice to dance. It denies the fact that woman can choose to be sexy and safe in that sexiness. It denies the fact that humans can overcome oppression – without having to give up their jobs. More seriously, it denies the fact that women are most at risk from abuse from people that they know. It denies the fact that women are raped and it is not talked about, because women shouldn't be sex objects.

It is a sinister ploy to detract from the real, enduring problems we have in society. It exacerbates the problem of thinking that 'lap dancers are this type of person' and the attitude of: 'Well I'm campaigning for them, for their happiness, yet for the most part I don't know them and I don't have a genuine dialogue with them.' It generalises problems that may be particular to that individual and require specific support. It demonises men who find women attractive – drives underground a very strong desire which, when suppressed, causes more problems to humanity than when openly admitted and discussed. The denial is always the problem; this is the real basis of addictive behaviour, in my (un-researched) opinion.

Yes, OK, there are things about the industry that I abhor. I abhor the fact that dancers are called 'self-employed' but are required to: a/ pay the club to dance there; b/ turn up at a particular time; and c/ abide by all their rules. But, the last supply-teaching job I had ripped me off just as much financially. I just need to change my karma.

Yes, the licensing laws may have a loop-hole, but that has already changed anyway. Let's not get too distracted by that point.

How important is it to a woman that she develop sexual prowess? It depends on the woman, I guess. I object to anything that refers to lap dancers as one homogenous group of people with the same views and the same issues, the same feelings, the same problems, the same aspiration, the same values, the same amount of blow-jobs, the same aspiration to self-denigration, the same limited range of life experience, the same level of desperation leading to the same level of manipulation. The same life.

It's OK to become offended when people presume that all black people are the same, but when it comes to lap dancers the rules change. My contention is that to talk about lap dancers in this way exacerbates the very problem by creating a dialogue of powerlessness for women. Women, (including lap dancers) are powerful people – any campaigns that treat them as victims also lock them into that role. Of course women are not sex objects, nor should they be the object of the rage of oppressed women. Actually, I've been treated with more respect whilst being overtly sexual and scantily-clad in a lap dancing club than I have been just walking down the street, or at school for that matter. At least when I'm in a club, if anything happens the bouncers are there to protect me. When I'm walking down the road, or when a young man at school makes an inappropriate comment, there is no one to be seen.

Really, though, I enjoy the dialogue with the young men at school. How come I can hold my own in that environment. How is it that I can educate and remain grounded when the lesson appears to have taken a turn for the worse? Exactly where is it that I learned those skills of understanding the nature of the man? Where is it, that these kind of dialogues became the norm, and oppression of both sexes became a non-starter? Where? Exactly where?

There are plenty of men out there who are not so confident on the sexual-activity front. What type of women really speaks to them, with any kind of confidence and knowledge? Does anyone bother?

What about other women who would so love to be free sexually, but have absolutely no chance of being so. Where are the lobbyists for those women, who are suffering silently? We must transcend differences, not exacerbate them. We must, if we are to be happy.

I am not a label. I am not my job. Who am I? How do I search for my soul? Through bold, courageous action.

You, wish to place a label on me. You, wish to oppress me. It cannot be, I am free. This is my essentiality. (Excuse the crudeness of the rhyme.)

So, when my university seminar lecturers came in for a dance, they were clearly impressed that they'd educated me so well and complimented me on my ability/agility in the job. Nice, I like that.

Another young teacher enters the club. We have a discussion about the fact that to be a teacher is to be asexual. Clearly, a job like this is required to readdress the balance.

One man decided to test me on my numeracy skills. How many angles in a circle? Infinite.

My discussions were not only about sex, they were about life, about everything. I'm sexual and I'm everything at the same time. They are just not mutually exclusive and nor should they be. Don't cut me up and put me into lots of little boxes — that's just sadism.

While people are embroiled in the pornography of judgement and the escapist, hedonistic view of morality, many real injustices are going unnoticed. For me, objectification is synonymous with judgement and original sin, and I don't buy either concept. Sorry. Not sorry at all.

So, that was my, not so short, rant. Being a lap dancer has enabled me to fulfil a part of me that had been oppressed for many years. If I were to work in a brothel, the same would apply. I did go for an 'interview' in a brothel, but there were lots of unhealthy sexual practices on the menu. Why do men want to sleep with prostitutes without a condom and pay more money for the pleasure? Interesting.

Just one more point: the whole tenuous link between lap dancing and sex trafficking. Me and a close friend of mine —

who used to work as a lap dancer — have said that we've not yet met a woman who has been forced into lap dancing in that way — not one, never.

So, the next time you frequent a dancing club, let some of my argument ring in your ear. Recognise that although you may not be engaging with the whole woman, that whole woman is there. Some are real businesswoman, so they won't be interested in the chat, just the same as in many other jobs, but the whole woman is there. There is no part of her that is missed out.

When you watch the pole dancing, admire the beauty and the sheer athleticism. Clearly you can have a look at her body too, but don't miss the whole person — you can't miss the whole person and the self-expression. Women are not objects, no matter how they are treated. Women are women and, no matter what they do, let's be really careful to respect them.

Let me be really careful to respect myself. Thank you.

Solicitor

I am a woman in my early 30s, and I am qualified as a solicitor. When I left university I worked as a temp. in the City for about a year, before getting a job in a solicitors' firm. I was 21 and excited, but naive. I thought it would be a great experience working in the City with these 'pillars of the community' – as I thought they were. The reality turned out to be very different.

Never have I been subject to so much sexism. Women were only there as objects to be looked at, commented on, and fawned over. All the office manager jobs were carried out by men, and the majority of administration work was done by women. There was a high turnover of administration and support staff, all temp. workers, and all women.

If there were drinks after work you had to be 'one of the lads' to fit in. In a supposedly professional environment, sexist jokes were banded around constantly, along with sexist and pornographic emails. The guys referred to their wives or girlfriends as 'her indoors' – something they could do without – and never as loved ones, partners, or even fellow human beings. They would go to strip clubs in their lunch breaks and not think anything of slapping my bottom as they walked past.

Why did I put up with it? Why did I not report it? Well, it was my first office job after university. I was also very shy, hated confrontation, and extremely naive. I had never encountered anything like this and inexperience can be disarming.

I then worked in various solicitors', and the blatant sexism continued. One Christmas party we went out for a meal. Straight after dessert was served, all the men in the office left to go to a strip club, with a few of the secretaries in tow, leaving the rest of us at the restaurant. One of the secretaries went simply because she was having an affair with one of the solicitors and wanted to check what he was getting up to. Another went to fit in 'with the lads' and seem cool. Only one man didn't go, and I have always respected him for not following the crowd.

I have had conversations with other women who hate the whole 'lad culture' in the office but, faced with such entrenched attitudes, it is not easy to bring this to your employers without suffering derision and further propagating the divide. My present employers know I am a strong feminist, and my feelings about strip clubs, and prostitution, are well known. However, even in what is a comparatively moderate environment, any discussion on these topics still serves only to distance me from the others, as it's still 'just a laugh' — nothing to be taken 'seriously'.

I feel I am sidelined, and I know I am talked about behind my back as the 'prudish, fun-hating' employee. Personally, this does makes me feel worthless.

I feel I am judged only by my appearance and not by my abilities. I have spoken to countless 'professional' men who only stare at my chest while talking to me; I have had comments about what I wear, my hair, my lack of makeup. It seems that it is perfectly acceptable to comment if I wear trousers more than skirts, or, if I do wear a skirt, I'm 'getting my legs out' for clients, or for the office. I am public property. I have never heard any similar comments being made to men.

Once the debate is opened, it has always surprised me how many other woman feel like this and are treated in exactly the same way.

Any organisation supporting women has a huge task ahead of them. Underlying sexism has become so ingrained that it is seen as entirely acceptable behaviour — just a bit of fun or a laugh. However, by opening up the debate and raising awareness, I hope people might start to think what is and is not acceptable office 'banter'. This has gone on too long.

Activist

'Women are being sold as cheaply as pints of beer! Only a fiver for a fully nude strip! What do YOU think about that?' This was how my involvement with OBJECT's lap dancing campaign began, during my first interview with OBJECT founder and director Dr Sasha Rakoff. I had previously met Sasha years before as a student volunteer for OBJECT, and now found myself nervously pitching for what seemed to be an exciting campaign to be involved with, despite the misgivings of the people close to me.

Although I didn't have much contact with feminism while I was growing up, I had long been aware of the weirdness that exists in our society around women, men and sexuality. As a schoolgirl I remember noticing the stares of men on the bus or in the street, and being aware that they were turned on by my looks and school uniform. It always left me with an uncomfortable feeling. Experiences such as this, and a desire to see a more peaceful world with less anger between all people, including between men and women, drew me towards OBJECT.

OBJECT's campaign to change the licensing of lap dancing clubs was already partially underway when I came onboard, and my mission was to pull together a national campaign. This campaign was eventually called 'Stripping the Illusion' (we were kindly granted permission by journalist Julie Bindel to use the name). We joined forces with the Fawcett Society and our target was to show the government that their choice to put lap dancing clubs in the same licensing category as 'leisure' venues — such as cafes, cinemas and pubs — flew in the face of what really occurs in lap dancing clubs.

I set about finding out for myself what 'really occurs in lap dancing clubs'. This involved sometimes strange experiences and meetings. The first time I tried to go to a club my colleague and I were refused entry because we were two women alone, with no men accompanying us. One of the clubs told us that it was too risky having women visit the club alone, as 'they often try to solicit the girls to work in their brothels'. When I asked what would stop men doing that, they didn't know what to say and we were told to return as part of a hen-night group.

For the campaign I met a variety of women who had worked in lap dancing clubs. If media depictions of lap dancing had been true, I would have met a whole host of hard-up students, living the 'sex, drugs and money' lifestyle. However, life is rarely that one-dimensional! I met women who had found their way into lap dancing for a whole multitude of reasons, and had different experiences; some were doing it part-time whilst others were working night after night in the clubs. What struck me early on in the campaign was that, despite these differences, key themes soon stood out from the testimonies I was collecting. All of the women I met complained about their treatment by club owners and the punters they danced for, with a lack of respect for their bodies, and 'self-value' emerging as a common theme. The disparity between glamorised and sanitised images of lap dancing and the more abusive reality of what they actually experienced in the private rooms and booths of the clubs they danced in, was talked about by every woman I met, as well as the difficulty of earning money given the working structure of most clubs.

One of the most surreal moments of the campaign involved sitting in a boardroom meeting of the Lap Dancing Association, a trade body that was created to help counter our campaign. Alongside my courageous colleague Kat Banyard, we walked into a small boardroom where a dozen club owners sat waiting for the meeting to begin. To say we stuck out like a sore thumb would be a bit of an understatement. After a somewhat eccentric short story about naval ships passing in the night – obviously code for 'we have two feminist intruders!' – we were asked to elaborate on our campaign before being shown the door 45 minutes later.

One of the arguments we heard at that meeting was that we should leave lap dancing clubs alone because they are isolated from society and have no effect on other women. However, I met women who felt scared to walk home at night because of clubs that had opened in their neighbourhoods; men who felt intimidated by the groups of men; as well as women whose relationships had totally changed after their partners had used the clubs. In my point of view this is hardly surprising. We don't live on isolated islands, totally separate from one another. Each action a person takes impacts on another, whether it be in thought, word or deed. What impact do lap dancing clubs have? If women living near a lap dancing club do not feel comfortable walking nearby a club after nightfall, can a club truly be said to have no impact on the rest of society?

And what also struck me was that neither party – the women working in the clubs, and the men using the clubs – seemed to be having a rewarding experience from their involvement with lap dancing. The portrayal of women and the relationship between men and women often felt so artificial that it reminded me of a scene in the film *The Matrix*, where the cliché of a beautiful women in a red dress is created by one of the characters. She appears real, available and wishing to attract men, but she is actually an illusion, created by a computer programme. How much of what we believe about lap dancing clubs is actually based on fantasy: the fantasy that it is a fun environment, that all women love working there, or that all men feel good when they are inside the clubs. And how much of what goes on in the clubs themselves is also closer to fantasy than reality?

Most of the women I met talked about the act they put on within the clubs, pretending to be foreign or 'dumbing down' their persona so as to appeal to the men buying lap dances. They said many of the men would similarly put on an act, passing themselves off as millionaires, airline pilots or budding entrepreneurs, when the women knew all too well this was far from the truth. If lap dancing clubs are marketed and believed to be a place where 'men can be men and women can be women', yet both are putting on acts, what does this say about our society and the relationship between men and women?

If I have one thing to say about the campaign now, two years later, I would ask what interactions between women and men would look like in a world where there was no judgement of what it means to be a woman and what it means to be a man? A world where the two could live side by side and enjoy each other. Call me a dreamer but I know that that world is possible, and I hope that, by creating more awareness, this will be achieved.

One of the things I enjoyed most about being part of the 'Stripping the Illusion' campaign was seeing how the issue brought together women and men from totally different backgrounds and perspectives, and how everyone worked side by side to create change regarding something they cared about. For example, at a meeting of volunteers in Brick Lane, London, we decided to sing songs at the campaign launch, and brainstormed songs together. I felt comfortable enough to brave a rap based on the catchy sounding 'Gender Equality Duty', which unsurprisingly never made it past draft stage! Moments like this remind me that when we come together, all sorts of things are possible, whether they be ridiculous raps or leglisative success! I'm really grateful for the experience of working on the campaign and to everyone involved. In the end we succeeded in changing the law. What else is possible?!

Part 2
ANALYSIS

Some background to the industry

Lap dancing, despite a high prevalence of clubs and establishments in the UK, is still a largely undocumented industry. Women performing for the sexual stimulation of paying male observers has a long history, from the Auletrides of Classical Greece, to the 'beautiful dancing girls' of central Asia – who as concubines were under absolute control of ruling emperors – to North American burlesque dancers of the post-World War Two period. Today, a contemporary offshoot of this tradition – the commercial strip club – as popularised in the US, has become big business with the rise of global strip club chains. In the United States the top thirty strip clubs are valued between $700 million and $1 billion alone,[1] with the total industry estimated to be worth $75 billion worldwide.[2] The UK's first official lap dancing club opened in north London in 1995. Prior to this other clubs existed that were not formal lap dancing clubs but combined dancing with nightclub or restaurant facilities, which allowed for a tentative licensing agreement.

As the industry has evolved, the nature and style of dancing available has changed. In the UK so called 'stripper nights' have been available since the 1960s in public houses, but at that time there was a stigma attached to watching women

---

[1] Sheerman 2007.
[2] Montgomery 2005.

stripping, and the practice was perceived as socially unacceptable. In the 1970s, public houses that held stripper activities had a policy in which customers were under no obligation to pay for watching a stripper; instead the dancer was expected to hand round a jug to collect tips. However, during the 1980s many venues stopped paying women altogether and instead began charging substantial 'stage fees'. Most performers now pay to work in strip clubs as 'independent contractors', who are nonetheless bound by fines or dismissal to a variety of rules and customs. Union attempts to reinstate wages instead of stage fees resulted in considerable opposition from club owners and some performers. To further increase profitability many clubs also began offering lap dancing, a form of striptease that involves performers sitting directly on a customer's lap and dancing against it. Today it is standard practice across the industry for dancers to pay a rent or house fee to the owner prior to working. Dancers may also have to pay additional money to the owner, usually a percentage from the money earned performing private dances, or even a percentage of tips.

Another major shift has involved the establishment of private 'VIP' rooms in which a consumer can experience a 'private' dance, as an alternative to the previously more common stage show. The average lap dancer will derive most of their income from performing private dances; often stage shows performed are for self-advertising purposes, and receiving a wage for performing on stage is not common practice. The majority of registered lap dance clubs in the UK now have such private facilities in which dancers make most of their income, but which are also the source of most of the controversy surrounding lap dancing.

The last two decades have seen concerted efforts by the industry to shake off its 'seedy' image by rebranding itself as high-class and glamorous. Many clubs now market themselves using the language of affluence and luxury, promoting their venues for corporate hospitality, charity fundraising and stag nights. The strategy appears to have paid off, as year on year more clubs have appeared in the UK. There are commentators who are concerned with this growth and argue that the rise of lap dancing clubs has led to an increase in human trafficking, rape and sexual assault, and the sexual-objectification of women.

Lap dancing clubs can be a lucrative business venture, generating money through a variety of sources. The sale of alcoholic drinks and an entrance fee for customers produce the same source of revenue as an ordinary nightclub, but increasingly lap dancing clubs earn a substantial amount of income from the dancers. As we have seen, technically dancers are self-employed and pay a house fee as well as a commission on each dance. They must abide by the clubs rules, with failure to do so ultimately resulting in dismissal.

A typical dancer could pay between £40 to £120 in house fees, and on average 10 to 25% commission on each dance. This could mean a dancer would need to perform 12 private dances at £10 each to make the house fee. But with 25% commission on each dance, she would only net £90, so in reality would need to perform 16 dances simply to make the house fee. She would then need to perform more private dances to make any profit. This excludes any personal expenses. Most clubs do not provide the dancers with refreshments, so a dancer may need to purchase their own drinks and also cover any travel expenses. In addition to this many clubs enforce fines on dancers. Reasons for fines include arriving late, inappropriate dress, arguing with customers and missing a stage show.

It is clear that lap dancing may not be as lucrative as a young woman may imagine. However, the 300 plus clubs across the UK have no difficulty in finding women to accept these work conditions, despite the fact that dancers are not eligible for paid holidays, insurance or even a guarantee of long-term employment. Why then are so many young women eagerly embarking on a career in lap dancing, and arguably beginning a career in the sex industry?

One point of view is that of Ariel Levy, author of the 2006 polemic, *Female Chauvinist Pigs, Women and The Rise of Raunch Culture*. For Levy, a female chauvinist pig (FCP) is a woman who embraces and participates in the objectification of women, and subsequent 'raunch culture', with the enthusiasm of a typical male chauvinist pig. Levy references lap dancing and stripping throughout her book and at one point suggests that the willingness to be involved in stripping may be a deluded form of feminism. 'In this new formulation of raunch feminism stripping is as valuable to elevating womankind as gaining an education or supporting rape victims. Throwing a party where women grind against each other in their underwear while fully clothed men watch them is suddenly part of the same project as marching on Washington for reproductive rights.'[3]

Levy suggests that while women reject the ignorant, stupid, male, sexist pig, '...the female chauvinist pig is given an exalted status; she is funny, she gets it, she does not mind cartoonish stereotypes of female sexuality. The FCP asks: Why worry about disgusting or degrading when you could be giving or receiving a lap dance yourself? Why beat them when you can join them?'[4] Levy's FCP concept suggests that women are not only entering lap dancing for the money, which is often the assumed reason, but also for the perceived 'empowerment' it can offer them. But lap dancing has been accused of creating and fuelling serious societal problems that far overshadow and outweigh any personal empowerment or self-affirmation an individual dancer may feel they have achieved.

Many lap dancers may not consider themselves to be sex workers or part of the sex industry, but critics insist that lap dancing, stripping, table dancing, etc. are in fact a part of the sex industry. Melissa Farley, a psychologist, states that there is no significant difference between porn stars and prostitutes, and that stripping is a form of prostitution.[5] Farley says that '... prostitution today is a toxic cultural product, which is

---

[3] Levy 2006.
[4] Ibid.
[5] Levy 2006.

to say that all women are socialised to objectify themselves in order to be desirable, to act like prostitutes, to act out the sexuality of prostitution'.[6]

Researcher and journalist Julie Bindel compiled a report for Glasgow council in 2004 entitled *Profitable Exploits: Lap Dancing in the UK*. The report suggests that the provision of licences to lap dancing clubs at the time provided a legalisation that expands the boundaries of the sex industry and causes women to become products of mass consumption.[7]

The report notes an explicit breach of license conditions. Ten dances were observed during a visit to a lap dancing venue. Every dancer, during their performances, displayed the inside of their genitalia by spreading their legs above the customers' heads. This seemed to be an established part of the routine. As one customer put it, 'What's the point of seeing a strip show and not getting a bit of fanny? The fun part is seeing her cunt. You can open *The Sun* if you just want tits.'[8] The dancers' regular display of their genitalia represented a patent breach of licensing conditions. The club under observation had a Music and Dancing Licence, and any such premises that are likely to have nude entertainments are all subject to a condition that disallows the displaying of the 'genital, urinary or excretory organs at any time while they are providing the service'.[9]

---

[6] Ibid.
[7] Bindel 2004.
[8] Ibid.
[9] Ibid.

The report highlighted how easily the culture in a lap dancing club can transform from a titillating, no-contact dance venue to a physical sex environment. One observer said, 'If a girl is having sex for £5, the other girls get really pissed off because they then have to do it for £5 ... and if one girl in a strip club is having sex, the others have to do it to make money'.[10]

Bindel asserted that her study has '... revealed the complex process and set of conditions in which dancers become more susceptible to requests or suggestions to sell sex. The lack of employment rights, for some women the experience of accumulating debt, expectations of the customers, fierce competition, and a link in public perceptions between lap dancer and stripper/prostitute, create an overall climate where the selling and buying of sex on the premises becomes more likely'.[11] Such behaviour observed within the clubs in this report challenges the contention that lap dancing is a harmless and legitimate part of the leisure industry.

From a broader perspective, the proliferation of lap dancing clubs can be seen to reflect the intense exploitation of sex in marketing, media and advertising, and the normalisation and integration of the sex industry into mainstream culture. In this context the current growth in lap dancing venues could be attributed to the prevalence of sexual content within mainstream society, demonstrating the effect of female

---

[10] Ibid.
[11] Ibid.

sexual objectification, in which every citizen plays a conscious or unconscious role.

There has been a storm raging over the licensing of lap dancing clubs. Since 2004, the year of Julie Bindel's aforementioned report, their number in the UK is believed to have doubled to over 300 active clubs.[12] Many believe that the licensing loophole that allowed lap dancing clubs to open under the same licence as cafes is behind this. Since April 2010, councils in England and Wales have been given new powers to control lap dancing clubs. The clubs will be classified as sex establishments and residents will be able to oppose venues for being 'inappropriate' to their area. Existing clubs have 12 months to apply for the new licence. Although hailed by many as a victory for those opposed to lap dancing clubs, councils have the right to apply this law in their area, and thus the impact of this new legislation is entirely in their hands. Lap dancing club owners have said that this change in the law will lead to job losses and lower investment in a 2.1 billion pound industry.[13]

---

[12] OBJECT 2009.
[13] BBC news website 2010.

Entertainment or Exploitation?

In many of the experiences in this book, a shift is acknowledged from what could tentatively be called a 'good club' or a 'good period of time for lap dancing' to what is frequently described as 'a bad time'. What changed? It could be reasonably argued that the growth in material of a sexual nature within modern media and marketing campaigns has had a marked effect on lap dancing clubs, particularly the working environment. Lap dancing clubs offering a topless or nude dancing service must now compete with various forms of media, such as DVDs, magazines and the internet, that provide equally — and often more gratuitously — sexual material to titillate the consumer. Access to explicit sexual content within the mainstream has led lap dancing clubs to compete by offering, increasingly, greater — and actual — sexual contact. This in turn has created a demand for greater sexuality within lap dancing clubs, and the dancers and the clubs have responded. Frequently, consumers now expect some form of sex to be offered via a lap dancing club and, as documented in the experiences in this book, openly object if this 'need' is not met.

Many social commentators believe the rise in sexual content within mainstream media and in the marketing of products and services is of great concern for additional reasons. Particularly alarming is the effect on young people.

In the past year there has been an outcry over products, such as padded-bras and T-shirts plastered with sexual innuendo, marketed at children and young people. In our society there are teenagers and young adults who are now displaying behaviour that reflects this sex-saturated culture. The aspiration of many young women to become 'glamour' models and lap dancers highlights the acceptance this generation has of the sex industry, but the rise in sexually-transmitted diseases in teenagers and young adults also indicates the naivety of these young people in understanding and experiencing sex.

Media and marketing material provide a one-dimensional viewpoint of sex, that claims to empower women in their lifestyle and career choices, whilst offering an increasingly warped vision of what sexuality is. As the sex industry is normalised, young people are, seemingly, having an increasingly unsafe understanding and a limited interpretation of sex.

In regard to lap dancing clubs, the UK government responded in 2010 by reclassifying the clubs as sex establishments, and therefore appears to have acknowledged the sexual nature of lap dancing. Campaigners who have striven for lap dancing clubs to be reclassified, in the light of the experiences shared in this book, appear to have had a valid point. The reclassification of the clubs provides a more transparent image of what they truly are, and ensures that consumers know what to expect. Residents in the vicinity now have a clearer picture of the nature of the club, and more importantly any new dancers, especially young women, have a clearer idea of the work they are undertaking. Under this new classification the dancer could be described as providing a sexual encounter, which has far more serious connotations than performing a 'lap dance'.

Why do women choose to work in this industry? Money and lifestyle expectations are conveyed as the key motivators and drivers for women to be involved; also, naive attitudes as to what being a lap dancer actually involves. The question as to whether lap dancing is part of the sex industry, and whether lap dancers are therefore sex workers, is one that may never be answered conclusively, due to the subjective definition of a sex worker. However, this book provides strong evidence that there has been a shift from what could reasonably be called 'lap dancing' to actual sexual encounters.

Ultimately, the experiences in this book have shown that the reality of lap dancing clubs in the UK is one characterised by, on the one hand, *sex*, and, on the other, *illusion*. The lap dancing industry claims to provide a fantasy for men, but the real fantasy is the lie on which the whole industry is based. Lap dancing is not a transparent profession. So far, little real information – apart from sensationalist documentaries and glamorised images – have been available. This is juxtaposed with a celebrity culture that is often fanatical about the perfect female body and idolises women who act in an explicitly sexual manner.

The industry has grown without many people having any

clear sense of the true reality and nature of the clubs. Researchers seem to have ignored the obvious people from whom one could gain real information – and from whom to understand the true reality of lap dancing – the actual dancers! This is largely due to the stereotypes that dehumanise dancers and ensure their silence, and also the secretive manner in which many dancers undertake their work. For a true documentation of the nature of lap dancing clubs, the dancers must be given the respect they deserve and a voice, because the reality is – however society tries to dismiss the dancers – they are providing a service this culture has demanded, and are a reflection of a 'generation sex' that people of today have created, participated in, and now appear largely to have accepted.

So what should be done about lap dancing clubs or, more correctly, sex establishments in the future? Would a ban of all clubs, enforced by the government, solve all the problems associated with lap dancing? Prohibition would provide a clear statement that lap dancing clubs, in all their forms, are unacceptable. However, an enforced ban would simply cut off an effect of a much deeper, more insidious, cause that exists in society. The UK is perceived, globally, to be a highly developed country, yet – decades since women received the vote and enjoyed the freedom provided by the contraceptive pill – one can observe a polarisation between men and women.

How is it still culturally acceptable for a fully-clothed man to pay a woman to strip naked in front of him, and often his friends, for the sole purpose of the male's gratification? And, for an aware woman to believe that this in some way empowers her? Lap dancing is not simply a feminist issue. It does not just oppress women. It humiliates us all. The belief that women make vast amounts of money providing this service seems to justify its existence and eliminates any argument of harm to the woman, and women in general. In a capitalist society that values economics and profit over all else, lap dancing does indeed appear to have a place. But, really, is this the best we as a society can do?

A way forward

Is this a hopeless situation? What can be done? It is, unde-
niably, very difficult to alter patterns of behaviour, especially
in adults; therefore the most constructive approach might be
to better educate future generations. I would propose that
secondary schools offer a more comprehensive form of sex
education, one that includes not just descriptions of biology,
but discussions of emotions, feelings and attitudes towards
sex. This education would have to include the wider social
implications of sex and sexuality, and discuss the use of lap
dancing and prostitution. Lap dancers, prostitutes and,
equally importantly, the men who will use these services in
the future, will be in that classroom. (Although women do use
the services of lap dancers and prostitutes, it is still pre-
dominantly men.)

We don't come into the world as fully formed adults. How
different would a person's decision to enter the sex industry
be if she or he were armed with knowledge of the reality of
this world? Such knowledge would not be taught by a child's
regular teacher, so that it is awkward and embarrassing, but
by an outside organisation, for at least a full day, each year, so
that all the issues could be explored in a comprehensive way
and in a safe environment. How different would Britain be if
secondary school-aged children were taught openly about
issues surrounding phenomena such as lap dancing and

prostitution, as well as violent sexual activity such as abuse and rape? This would be balanced by encouraging healthy attitudes to sex; that masturbation is normal, as is homosexuality, and so on. These are very human issues that affect us all. Life is to be cherished, protected and enjoyed, not humiliated and destroyed through ignorance, power-mongering, fear and violence. Young people are wise enough to learn these lessons. Are we wise enough to teach them?

About OBJECT

OBJECT is an award-winning human rights organisation which challenges the sexual objectification of women and the mainstreaming of the sex and porn industries through lads' mags, lap dancing clubs or prostitution. OBJECT does this because of the attitudes these industries promote about women and the impact these beliefs and behaviours have on discrimination and violence against women.

OBJECT launched the 'Stripping the Illusion' campaign in 2008 to strip the illusion that lap dancing clubs are harmless fun. Lap dancing clubs normalise the sexual objectification of women, create 'no-go' zones for women, and are a form of commercial sexual exploitation. Yet until April 2010, lap dancing clubs in England and Wales were licensed in the same way as cafes and restaurants — as if they were an ordinary part of the leisure industry. This lax licensing served as a green light to the industry, which doubled in size in five years, despite mounting opposition from women's organisations and residents.

OBJECT launched a two-year campaign with the Fawcett Society and, with the help and support of trade and student unions, women who had worked in lap dancing clubs, feminist policy-makers, sister organisations and committed activists across the country, this culminated in a change to the law so that local councils can now license lap dancing clubs as sex establishments, not leisure venues. This law change gives councils greater powers to regulate the industry and allows for gender equality issues to be at the heart of the licensing debate. OBJECT is currently supporting local people to lobby their councils to ensure that this new legislation is used effectively.

An important part of the 'Stripping the Illusion' campaign has been to provide a platform from which women who have had negative experiences in the lap dancing industry can have their voices heard. From the beginning of the campaign, OBJECT worked in partnership with many women who painted a very different picture of the industry than the glamorised version peddled by the media. OBJECT made a film of video testimonies to expose these harsh realities and, in partnership with women's organisation Trust, has recently set up a support network for women who have had harmful experiences in the lap dancing industry, to be able to process common experiences in an environment which is non-judgemental, supportive and empowering.

For more information about any of the OBJECT campaigns, see the OBJECT website at www.object.org.uk

Acknowledgements

Thank you to my beautiful husband Hiro for his eternal love and support, and thank you to my mentor Daisaku Ikeda for all his guidance and wisdom. All my love to Lisa, Adele and Fran for their loyalty and care. Many thanks to Dr Anthony Patterson for his encouragement, Rob Wilson for his support, JB for teaching me to be strong no matter what, and Martin Barron and Chinapa Aguh for being there and not judging me when I finally 'came out'! Lots of love to Sandrine Lévêque and everyone at OBJECT. Sincere gratitude to Sevak Gulbekian and all those involved at Clairview Books for giving both this book and me a chance. Thank you to all the beautiful women who had the courage to contribute to this book. And finally, thank you to my parents and sister for giving me the space to make my own mistakes, never saying I told you so, and the opportunity to attempt to rectify those mistakes.

References

Barton, Bernadette (2006) *Stripped: Inside the Lives of Exotic Dancers*, New York: NYU Press

BBC News (2010) 'New powers to crack down on lap dancing clubs' URL: http://news.bbc.co.uk/1/hi/uk/8511883.stm

Bindel (2004) 'Profitable Exploits: Lap Dancing in the UK' URL: www.rapecrisisscotland.org.uk/documents/ profitable%20exploits.pdf

Brown, Louise (2005) *The Dancing Girls of Lahore*, New York, HarperCollins Publishers

Burana, Lily (2001) *Strip City: A Stripper's Farewell Journey Across America*, New York: Talk Miramax Books

Gill, Rosalind (2008) Speech given at Stripping the Illusion OBJECT Campaign Launch, House of Commons 22/04/08 [In possession of author]

Jeffreys, Sheila (2008a) 'The Strip Club Boom', chapter from *The Industrial Vagina: The Political Economy of the Global Sex Trade*, Routledge

Levy (2006) *Female Chauvinist Pigs: Women and the Rise of Raunch Culture*, London: Pocket Books

Montgomery, Dave (2005) 'Industry Trying to Take Its Image Upscale'. *Fort Worth Star-Telegram*, October 3. URL: http://www.accessmylibrary.com/coms2/summary_0286-9666939_ITM

Object (2009) URL: http://www.object.org.uk/

Ross, Becki; Kim Greenwell (2005) 'Spectacular Striptease: Performing the Sexual and Racial Other in Vancouver, B.C 1945–1975', *Journal of Women's History*, Vol. 17 No. 1 pp. 137–163

Sherman, William 2007. 'The Naked Truth about Strip Clubs'. *New York Daily News*, 08/10/08 URL: http://www.nydailynews.com

UK Lap (2008) *History of lap dancing* URL: http://www.uklap.com/history